MW01656961

Super Easy
HIGH PROTEIN

Low Carb Diet Cookbook for Beginners

Healthy, Delicious, Time-Saving Recipes to Build Strength, Burn Fat, Crush Cravings, and Keep Your Family Happy!

Mark L. Landers

Table of Contents

Introduction

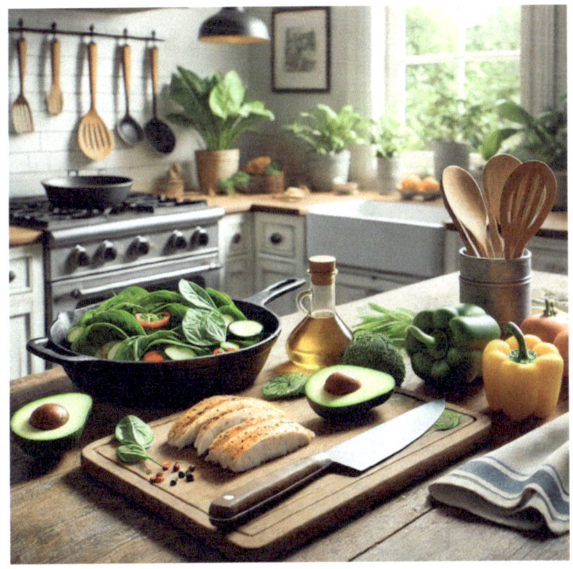

Many embark on the journey toward better health armed with hope but quickly find themselves overwhelmed by confusing advice, fleeting motivation, and unsustainable methods. The struggle is not just about losing weight or improving energy levels; it's about reclaiming control in a world designed to derail even the best intentions. A low-carb, high-protein strategy isn't just another diet—it's a scientifically grounded, practical approach to transforming not only your body but also your mindset.

For years, the nutritional narrative centered on calorie counting and restrictive eating, leaving people frustrated and caught in an endless cycle of crash diets. These plans often fail to address the root of the problem: fluctuating energy, persistent cravings, and hormonal imbalances caused by excessive carbohydrate consumption. A shift to this balanced approach breaks this cycle by targeting the physiological barriers to success, emphasizing satiety, metabolic harmony, and long-term feasibility.

Imagine mornings where you wake up refreshed, your mind sharp and your body revitalized, no longer weighed down by the sluggishness of sugar crashes or the emotional swings of carb-laden meals. Instead of grappling with hunger throughout the day, you feel nourished and in control, empowered by meals that align with your aspirations. This isn't just wishful thinking; it's the natural result of prioritizing high-quality proteins and low-glycemic foods in your daily life.

The beauty of this lifestyle lies in its adaptability. Unlike rigid, one-size-fits-all plans, it enables you to create a way of eating that reflects your unique preferences and schedule. Whether you're a busy parent juggling family responsibilities, a professional navigating hectic workdays, or someone striving for a healthier connection with food, this method integrates effortlessly into your routine. There's no need for deprivation or monotony—just a focus on satisfying, nutrient-dense meals that bring joy to every bite.

This nutritional philosophy tackles the modern challenge of overabundance with a transformative perspective. The prevalence of processed, carbohydrate-heavy foods has made it all too easy to consume empty calories, leading to inconsistent energy levels and compromised health. By focusing on nutrient-packed ingredients, this approach rewrites the narrative entirely. Lean proteins, healthy fats, and vibrant vegetables take center stage, not only reducing carbohydrate intake but also delivering the sustenance your body needs for peak performance and overall vitality.

The initial adjustment can feel intimidating—after all, change is never entirely comfortable. You might worry about letting go of your go-to comfort foods or navigating social settings. But here's the truth: embracing a low-carb, high-protein lifestyle isn't about restriction; it's about liberation. It's about breaking free from the cycle of cravings and energy dips, rediscovering the pleasure of guilt free eating, and feeling empowered in your own skin.

What makes this journey even more rewarding is the solid scientific foundation supporting it. Research consistently demonstrates that reducing carbohydrates while emphasizing protein-rich foods not only supports weight management but also improves markers of metabolic health, stabilizes blood sugar, and sharpens cognitive function. These benefits aren't short-lived; they serve as the foundation for a healthier, more vibrant future. Each time you opt for a nourishing, protein-rich meal, you're investing in yourself—in your energy, focus, and overall resilience.

This dietary approach isn't a fleeting fix or a temporary measure. It's a commitment to yourself, one that becomes increasingly intuitive with time. As you adapt, you'll notice how decisions that once seemed difficult—skipping the breadbasket or choosing grilled chicken over pasta—become instinctive. The changes will manifest not only in how you look but also in how you feel, day after day.

As you move forward, focus on progress rather than perfection. Small, steady adjustments lead to profound and lasting transformations. Adopting this mindset allows you to honor both your body and your goals. It's an opportunity to redefine your vision of health and create a life that reflects your fullest potential.

The journey begins with a single, empowering decision: to nourish your body and mind with intention. The chapters ahead will provide more than just recipes—they will offer insights and strategies to make this lifestyle a lasting and fulfilling part of your life. Together, we'll turn obstacles into opportunities, transforming your connection with food into one of balance and empowerment. Welcome to the first step of your transformation.

The Basics of the LCHP Diet

What Does "Low Carb" Mean?

At its core, a "low carb" approach is about minimizing the intake of carbohydrates in your daily diet. Carbohydrates, often referred to as "carbs," are a primary source of energy for the body, but not all are created equal. They come in various forms, ranging from simple sugars like glucose to complex ones found in foods like grains, vegetables, and legumes. In a low-carb diet, the focus is on drastically reducing the consumption of high-glycemic options such as refined sugars, white bread, and processed foods, while promoting nutrient-dense sources like leafy greens, cruciferous vegetables, and low-sugar fruits.

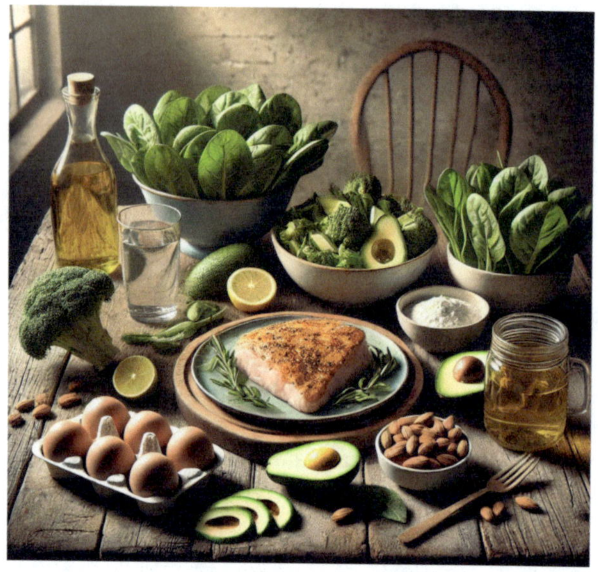

Why reduce carbs? When consumed in excess, carbohydrates are broken down into glucose, which enters the bloodstream, increasing blood sugar levels. In response, the body releases insulin, a hormone that helps cells absorb glucose. However, consistently high insulin levels can lead to fat storage, energy crashes, and, over time, insulin resistance. By cutting down on carbohydrates, the body adjusts its metabolic processes. With fewer carbs to use as fuel, it begins to depend more heavily on fat stores, a process known as ketosis or fat adaptation. This metabolic state not only supports weight loss but also provides steady, long-lasting energy throughout the day.

Reducing carbohydrates also has a profound impact on hunger and appetite. High-carb foods, particularly those with a high glycemic index, cause spikes in blood sugar followed by rapid drops. These fluctuations can trigger cravings and overeating. In contrast, a low-carb diet helps stabilize blood sugar levels, reducing hunger pangs and fostering a more controlled relationship with food.

Another key advantage of reducing carbs is its positive effect on overall health. Numerous studies have shown that a low-carb diet can improve markers of metabolic well-being, including better blood sugar control, lower triglycerides, and increased HDL ("good") cholesterol levels. These benefits make this dietary approach an attractive option for individuals aiming to not only lose weight but also enhance their long-term health and vitality.

Why "High Protein"?

While reducing carbs is essential, the "high protein" component of the diet is equally transformative. Proteins are the building blocks of life, made up of amino acids that play a crucial role in nearly every function of the body. Protein is essential for immune system support, tissue repair, and hormone synthesis. But what makes it so effective in a diet focused on weight management and overall health?

First and foremost, protein is a satiety powerhouse. Unlike carbohydrates or fats, protein takes longer to digest, providing a lasting feeling of fullness. This lessens the chance of overindulging and consuming harmful snacks. Studies have consistently shown that high-protein diets help regulate appetite hormones, including increasing levels of peptide YY, which signals fullness, and reducing levels of ghrelin, the hunger hormone. As a result, meals rich in protein leave you feeling satisfied for longer periods, making it easier to adhere to your dietary goals.

Moreover, protein has a unique property known as the "thermic effect of food" (TEF). This is the amount of energy your body uses to break down, absorb, and process food. Protein has the highest TEF of all macronutrients, meaning your body burns more calories processing protein than it does carbs or fats. This makes protein not only essential for muscle repair and growth but also an ally in boosting your metabolism and supporting fat loss.

High-protein diets are particularly effective in preserving lean muscle mass during weight loss. When you cut calories, there's a risk that your body will break down muscle for energy along with fat. By consuming sufficient protein, you provide your body with the amino acids it needs to maintain muscle, even in a calorie deficit. Maintaining muscle mass is essential because, as metabolically active tissue, muscle burns more calories at rest than fat. The more lean muscle you have, the higher your resting metabolic rate, and the easier it becomes to maintain a healthy weight over the long term.

In addition to its role in metabolism and muscle preservation, protein is incredibly versatile in the kitchen. A diet high in protein opens the door to a wide variety of delicious and satisfying meals. From grilled chicken and salmon to plant-based options like tofu and tempeh, the possibilities are nearly endless. The inclusion of protein in every meal not only supports your dietary goals but also adds texture and flavor to your dishes, making healthy eating an enjoyable experience rather than a chore.

Another important consideration is protein's role in overall health and wellness. Beyond weight loss and muscle maintenance, a high-protein diet supports stronger bones, enhanced immune function, and improved recovery from physical activity. For those with active lifestyles, protein is essential in repairing the micro-tears in muscle fibers caused by exercise, allowing for faster recovery and improved performance over time.

It's also worth noting that high-protein diets are highly adaptable. Whether you're an athlete looking to optimize performance, a professional aiming for steady energy throughout the day, or someone seeking weight loss, protein can be tailored to fit your specific needs. The key is to include high-quality sources of protein, such as lean meats, fish, eggs, dairy, and plant-based alternatives, while balancing portion sizes to align with your goals.

This balanced interplay between lowering carbs and increasing protein intake is the secret to unlocking a diet that not only supports your fitness and weight-loss goals but also fosters a sense of vitality and long-term health.

The Benefits of the LCHP Diet

Natural and Sustainable Fat Loss

One of the most compelling aspects of the Low Carb High Protein (LCHP) diet is its ability to facilitate natural and sustainable fat loss. Unlike extreme dieting trends that promise rapid results but are difficult to maintain, this approach works harmoniously with the body's natural processes, ensuring long-term success without feelings of deprivation or exhaustion.

The diet accelerates fat loss by reducing the intake of carbohydrates, forcing the body to shift its energy source from glucose to fat. This process, often referred to as "fat adaptation," triggers the breakdown of stored fat into molecules called ketones, which the body uses as an alternative fuel. With a steady, reduced supply of carbohydrates, your body becomes a highly efficient fat-burning machine, leveraging its reserves to power daily activities.

Low-carb eating promotes stable blood sugar levels, effectively eliminating the insulin spikes and crashes tied to high-carb diets. This approach helps control insulin, a hormone essential for glucose metabolism that also triggers fat storage. Consistently low insulin levels reduce fat accumulation, paving the way for steady weight loss. Beyond the physical transformation, this method fosters a sense of balance and renewed energy, reinforcing your drive to maintain the lifestyle.

Maintaining Lean Muscle Mass

Preserving lean muscle during weight loss is one of the key challenges people face with many traditional diets. Since muscle is metabolically active, it burns more calories while at rest than fat. Losing muscle not only slows down your metabolism but can also lead to feelings of weakness and fatigue. This is where the high-protein component of the diet plays a pivotal role.

Protein delivers the vital amino acids required for muscle repair and maintenance. During a calorie deficit, which is an inherent aspect of most weight-loss diets, the body often seeks muscle tissue as an alternative energy source. Consuming adequate protein ensures your body has the resources to safeguard muscle mass while effectively utilizing fat stores for energy.

In fact, high-protein diets have been shown to promote a more favorable body composition. Research consistently demonstrates that individuals on high-protein, low-carb diets tend to lose more fat while retaining or even gaining lean muscle mass compared to those on low-protein diets. This is particularly important for those who engage in regular exercise, as protein supports recovery and muscle repair after workouts.

Additionally, maintaining lean muscle mass has aesthetic benefits. As fat is reduced, the underlying muscle gives the body a toned and sculpted appearance, enhancing overall physical fitness and confidence. It's a transformative process that goes beyond the numbers on the scale, focusing instead on how you look and feel in your own skin.

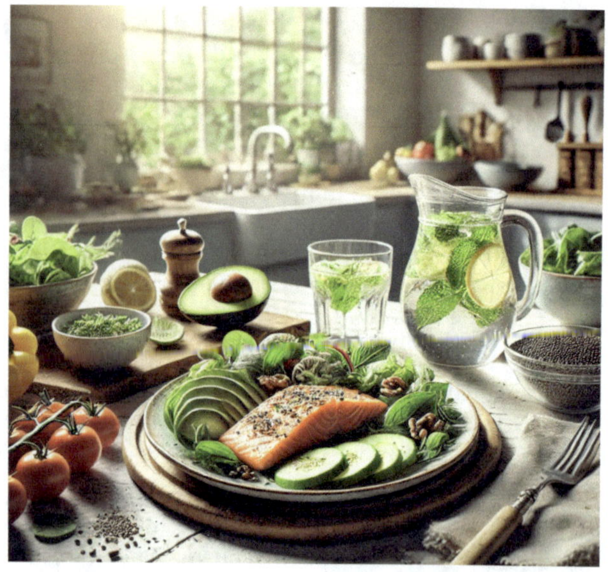

A Two-Pronged Approach to Effective Weight Loss

The combination of fat loss and muscle preservation is what sets this diet apart from many other weight-loss strategies. When you lose weight quickly on a crash diet, much of that loss often comes from water and muscle mass, leaving you weaker and more likely to regain the weight. This approach, on the other hand, ensures that the weight you lose is primarily fat, while your muscle mass remains intact. This dual action creates a positive cycle: as your body sheds fat, your metabolic rate stays high due to the preservation of muscle. You feel stronger, more energetic, and more capable of sticking to the diet long-term. This sustainability is crucial for achieving lasting results.

Appetite Control and Craving Reduction

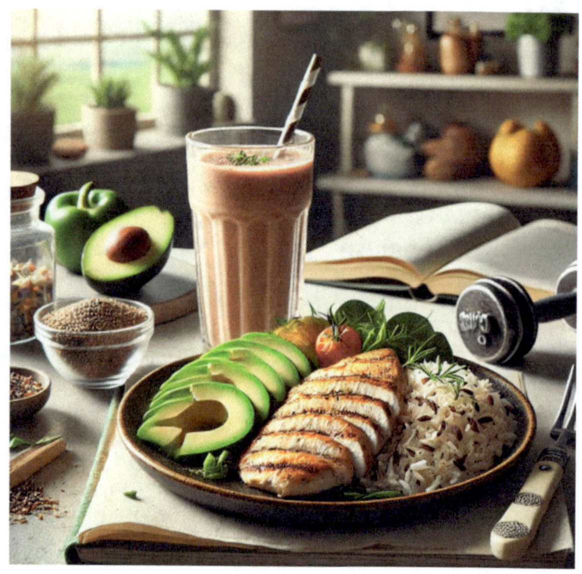

The diet excels at promoting sustainable fat loss largely due to its natural ability to regulate appetite. Protein's exceptional satiating properties ensure you remain satisfied for longer periods compared to meals dominated by carbohydrates or fats. Incorporating high-protein foods into every meal helps curb overeating and reduces the temptation of unhealthy snacking, making it easier to stay aligned with your health goals.

In addition to providing satiety, high-protein meals stabilize appetite hormones. Protein has been shown to increase levels of peptide YY, a hormone that signals fullness, while simultaneously reducing levels of ghrelin, the "hunger hormone." This hormonal balance makes it easier to adhere to your dietary goals without constantly battling cravings.

Low-carb eating effectively helps control hunger by stabilizing blood sugar levels. High-carb foods, especially those with a high glycemic index, lead to rapid blood sugar spikes followed by sharp drops, which often result in cravings for sugary or starchy options. Eliminating these foods from your diet breaks this cycle and fosters consistent energy throughout the day.

Long-Term Weight Maintenance

Another significant advantage of the LCHP diet is its effectiveness in preventing weight regain, a common problem with other dieting methods. Many people lose weight on restrictive diets, only to gain it back when they return to their usual eating habits. This approach, however, focuses on building habits that are both effective and sustainable.

The method prioritizes whole, nutrient-dense foods and satisfying meals, naturally reducing the appeal of returning to less nutritious choices. High-quality protein plays a vital role in preserving muscle mass and maintaining a strong metabolism, simplifying long-term weight management. Additionally, the diet's emphasis on balanced blood sugar and insulin levels fosters a hormonal balance that actively prevents fat accumulation.

For long-term success, the key is consistency rather than perfection. It is flexible enough to accommodate occasional indulgences, provided they are balanced by a return to low-carb, high-protein meals. This adaptability makes it a realistic and achievable lifestyle choice rather than a temporary fix.

Enhanced Fat-Burning Through Exercise

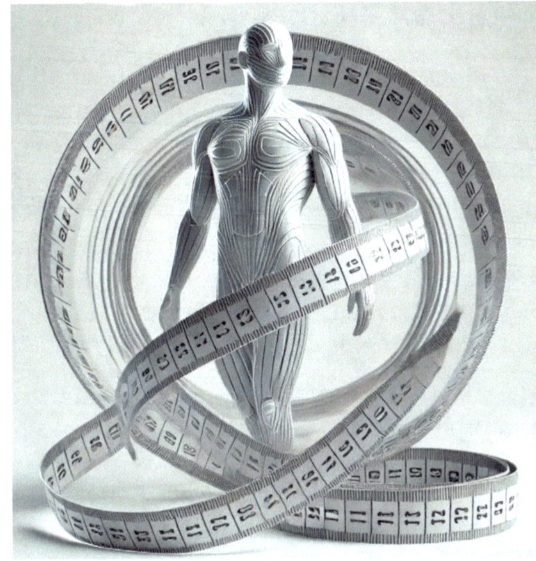

While the diet is effective on its own, its results can be amplified when combined with regular physical activity. Exercise, particularly resistance training, complements the approach by further promoting muscle retention and fat loss. The high protein intake supports recovery and muscle repair, making it easier to incorporate challenging workouts into your routine.

For those seeking maximum results, combining the diet with strength training creates a powerful synergy. As you build lean muscle, your body burns more calories at rest, accelerating fat loss and enhancing your overall physique. Even moderate activity, such as walking or yoga, can amplify the benefits by increasing energy expenditure and improving overall well-being.

The Low Carb High Protein diet is a holistic approach to achieving natural and sustainable weight loss. It emphasizes tapping into fat reserves, preserving muscle mass, and managing hunger effectively, providing a streamlined path to reaching your health goals. This journey isn't just about appearance—it's about feeling empowered, energized, and ready to embrace life with renewed confidence.

Enhanced Energy and Mental Focus

The diet goes beyond physical transformation, offering a foundation for sustained energy and mental empowerment throughout the day. Its ability to stabilize blood sugar levels creates the ideal conditions for improved focus and sharper cognitive function, making it a powerful choice for enhancing productivity and mental clarity.

At the core of this transformation lies the role of carbohydrates—or rather, their strategic reduction. High-carb meals, especially those loaded with refined sugars or processed grains, lead to rapid spikes in blood sugar. While these spikes may temporarily boost energy, they are inevitably followed by crashes that leave you feeling sluggish, unfocused, and irritable. In contrast, this approach maintains steady blood sugar levels by prioritizing low-glycemic vegetables and healthy protein sources. This stability ensures a consistent supply of energy to the brain, which thrives on a reliable flow of fuel. The result? A clearer, sharper mind that is better equipped to handle complex tasks, make decisions, and stay focused for extended periods.

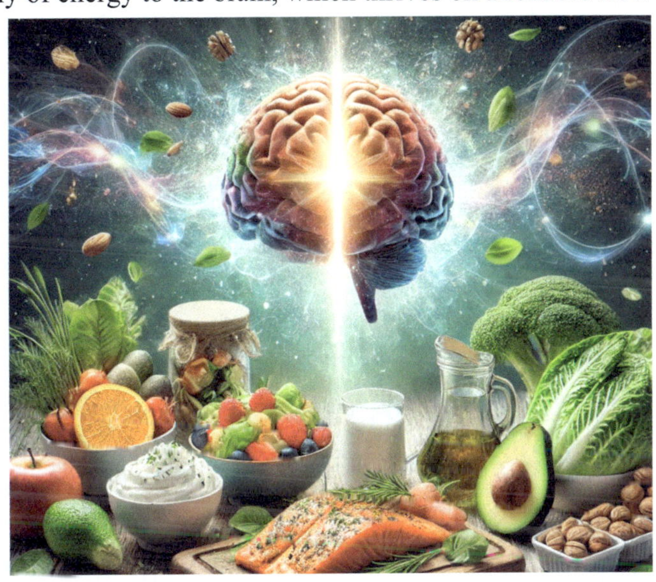

Proteins play a complementary role in this cognitive uplift. As the building blocks of neurotransmitters—the chemical messengers of the brain—proteins influence mood, memory, and concentration. Foods rich in protein, such as eggs, fish, or lean meats, provide the amino acids necessary for producing dopamine and serotonin. These neurotransmitters are essential for maintaining motivation, focus, and an overall sense of well-being. Moreover, protein's ability to sustain energy levels through its slow digestion adds another layer of support to maintaining mental sharpness throughout the day.

Enhanced concentration depends not only on nourishing the brain but also on reducing physical discomfort and fatigue that can divert attention. This dietary strategy effectively prevents mid-morning or mid-afternoon energy crashes, often linked to a craving for sugary foods, by ensuring prolonged satiety. With hunger pangs and cravings no longer disrupting your day, it becomes easier to stay fully engaged in your work, studies, or creative pursuits.

The benefits of blood sugar stability extend beyond mental focus. A balanced diet that reduces insulin spikes creates a harmonious environment within your body, reducing the inflammation and oxidative stress often linked to diets high in processed carbs. This internal equilibrium supports not only brain health but also long-term resilience against cognitive decline. It's a lifestyle change that primes you for success today while safeguarding your mental clarity for the years to come.

Sustained Stamina for the Entire Day

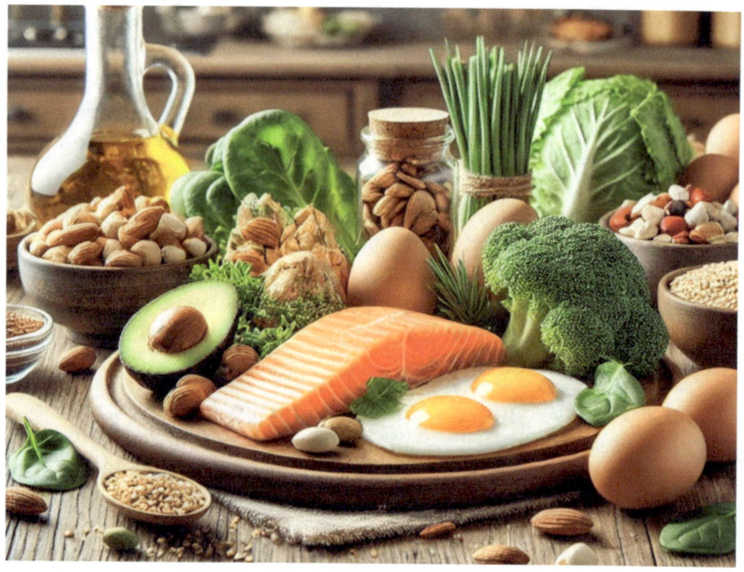

One of the most noticeable effects of transitioning to an LCHP diet is the steady stream of energy it provides. Unlike traditional high-carb diets, which can leave you riding a rollercoaster of energy highs and lows, the low-carb approach offers a more consistent and reliable source of vitality. This is particularly important for people with demanding schedules, from professionals balancing meetings to parents chasing after children, or athletes seeking peak performance.

The main source of energy for the body is adenosine triphosphate (ATP), which is made from macronutrients such as proteins, lipids, and carbs. When you reduce carbohydrates in your diet, your body becomes more efficient at using fat as a fuel source. This metabolic shift, often referred to as fat adaptation, enables a longer-lasting energy supply. Fat is a denser source of energy compared to carbohydrates, and its slower rate of metabolism means you avoid the quick bursts and sudden crashes that characterize sugar-fueled energy. This steady release ensures that you remain energized from morning to night without the need for constant snacking or caffeine boosts.

High protein intake also plays a crucial role in maintaining endurance. Proteins, while not typically the body's primary energy source, support muscle function and recovery, which are key to sustaining physical stamina. Whether you're climbing stairs, running errands, or engaging in vigorous exercise, the amino acids derived from protein-rich foods repair muscle fibers and reduce the fatigue associated with daily wear and tear. Over time, this translates to greater physical resilience and the ability to sustain a higher level of activity without feeling drained.

Moreover, the combination of low-carb and high-protein eating supports optimal hydration levels, which are often disrupted by carb-heavy diets. Carbohydrates bind to water in the body, so as you reduce your intake, you shed excess water weight. While this initially leads to a drop in water retention, it encourages you to hydrate more effectively with electrolyte-rich fluids. Proper hydration enhances circulation, ensures efficient oxygen delivery to tissues, and keeps energy levels robust throughout the day.

For those integrating exercise into their routine, this lifestyle delivers unparalleled benefits. As the body transitions to burning fat for fuel, it taps into a virtually inexhaustible energy reserve, making it ideal for sustained endurance activities. Unlike glycogen, which depletes relatively quickly during prolonged exertion, fat stores provide a consistent and reliable energy source. Additionally, the high-protein focus ensures effective muscle recovery and repair, leaving you stronger and ready to face your next challenge with confidence.

Metabolic Health

The Low Carb High Protein diet significantly enhances metabolic health, presenting itself as a transformative solution for optimizing overall well-being. This nutritional strategy ensures peak bodily efficiency through a focus on stabilizing blood sugar levels and mitigating the risks associated with chronic diseases.

At the heart of this diet is its ability to stabilize blood sugar levels. Lowering carbohydrate intake causes the body's glucose levels to rise and fall less frequently. This stability is essential, as erratic blood sugar can lead to fatigue, cravings, and over time, insulin resistance. Insulin, the hormone responsible for helping cells absorb glucose, plays a pivotal role here. When consistently high levels of insulin are required to manage frequent glucose surges, the body can become less responsive, a condition known as insulin resistance. This is often a precursor to type 2 diabetes and other metabolic disorders.

This dietary approach naturally reduces the body's reliance on insulin through a strategic focus on minimizing carbohydrate intake while emphasizing proteins and healthy fats. This fosters a more stable metabolic state, enhances the body's ability to utilize energy efficiently, and lowers the likelihood of developing chronic complications. For individuals dealing with blood sugar-related conditions, this framework offers an effective, non-invasive solution that can improve overall quality of life while potentially reducing the need for extensive medication.

Proteins play a critical role in supporting metabolic health. Foods rich in protein have a minimal impact on blood sugar levels, avoiding the sharp spikes often caused by other macronutrients. Additionally, protein enhances the thermic effect of food (TEF), which refers to the energy your body expends during digestion and metabolism. Consuming higher amounts of protein boosts calorie-burning capacity even at rest, improving metabolic efficiency while aiding in effective weight management.

Another remarkable benefit of this diet is its impact on lipid profiles. Chronic intake of refined carbs and sugars has been shown to elevate triglycerides and reduce HDL (the "good" cholesterol), two markers associated with an increased risk of cardiovascular disease. By reducing carbohydrate consumption, it naturally lowers triglycerides while promoting the production of HDL. This balance is crucial for maintaining heart health and reducing the likelihood of atherosclerosis or other cardiovascular complications.

The focus on nutrient-dense, low-carb foods such as leafy greens and lean proteins brings a wealth of essential vitamins, minerals, and antioxidants to your plate. These powerful micronutrients work to reduce inflammation and combat oxidative stress—two critical factors that fuel metabolic conditions and chronic disease. Embracing this lifestyle, with its emphasis on whole, unprocessed foods, becomes a proactive step toward safeguarding your health and slowing the progression of disease.

Reduced Risk of Chronic Diseases

The link between diet and chronic disease is undeniable, and the LCHP diet stands out as a proactive strategy for minimizing the risk of serious health conditions. One of its most notable benefits is its capacity to help prevent type 2 diabetes. By stabilizing blood sugar levels and enhancing insulin sensitivity, this approach tackles key factors that contribute to the disease. Excessive insulin production, a primary driver of diabetes, is mitigated through the careful avoidance of high-glycemic foods, making this dietary framework both practical and impactful.

In addition to its benefits for diabetes prevention, this diet supports cardiovascular health. Elevated blood pressure, another hallmark of metabolic syndrome, often improves with the adoption of a low-carb diet. This effect can be attributed to the reduction in water retention and inflammation that accompanies a decrease in carbohydrate consumption. Paired with the improved lipid profiles seen in many individuals, these changes significantly lower the risk of heart attacks, strokes, and related complications.

The diet's anti-inflammatory properties contribute to its ability to protect against a variety of chronic conditions. Autoimmune disorders and degenerative diseases, including rheumatoid arthritis and Alzheimer's, are often exacerbated by persistent inflammation. Reducing the intake of processed foods and carbohydrate-rich options that fuel inflammatory responses helps create a physiological environment less conducive to the progression of these illnesses. Pairing omega-3-rich foods like walnuts and fatty fish with antioxidant-packed vegetables further amplifies these protective effects, promoting cellular health and supporting long-term vitality.

Cancer prevention is another area where this approach shows promise. While no diet can eliminate the risk entirely, reducing sugar intake is increasingly recognized as a step toward decreasing cancer risk. Many cancer cells thrive on glucose; thus, a diet that limits glucose availability can theoretically slow the growth of these cells. Additionally, the focus on whole foods and lean proteins minimizes exposure to harmful additives and preservatives often linked to cancer.

Mental health, often overlooked in discussions of chronic disease, also benefits from this dietary approach. Emerging research suggests that diets high in processed carbohydrates and sugars may contribute to the onset of depression and anxiety through mechanisms involving inflammation and gut health. The emphasis on protein and healthy fats helps support the production of neurotransmitters like serotonin and dopamine, which are essential for mood regulation. This dietary approach also promotes a balanced gut microbiome, a factor increasingly linked to both physical and mental health.

The long-term adherence to this lifestyle is facilitated by its holistic approach to nourishment. Unlike restrictive fad diets, it emphasizes the inclusion of satisfying, flavorful foods that meet your body's needs for macronutrients and micronutrients alike. This sustainability not only enhances compliance but also ensures that the benefits for metabolic health and chronic disease prevention are maintained over the years, contributing to a longer, healthier life.

General Well-Being: A Holistic Transformation

The Low Carb High Protein diet has transformative effects not only on weight and energy levels but also on broader aspects of well-being. Adopting this lifestyle can result in a radiant complexion, improved sleep patterns, and a more stable, positive mood. These benefits stem from the diet's ability to nourish the body with essential nutrients while eliminating the inflammatory and disruptive impacts of processed carbohydrates and sugars.

One of the most striking transformations that come with this diet is the noticeable improvement in skin's radiance and health. High-carb diets, particularly those rich in refined sugars, are infamous for triggering inflammation and glycation—two processes that break down collagen and elastin, the proteins essential for maintaining skin's firmness and elasticity. By shifting the focus to nutrient-dense proteins and healthy fats while significantly reducing carbohydrate intake, this dietary approach helps mitigate such damage. The outcome is a complexion that appears healthier, smoother, and more luminous, with fewer instances of redness or breakouts. On top of that, the emphasis on hydration, combined with the reduced water retention that often accompanies lower carbohydrate consumption, works synergistically to refine skin clarity and amplify its natural glow.

Proteins and healthy fats, staples of this diet, also play a vital role in supporting skin health. Proteins provide the amino acids necessary for collagen production, ensuring the skin remains firm and youthful. Fats, particularly those rich in omega-3 fatty acids found in fish, nuts, and seeds, combat dryness and inflammation, enhancing the skin's barrier function and natural glow. These combined effects create a noticeable improvement in skin quality over time, giving you the confidence that comes with looking and feeling your best.

The benefits of the diet extend beyond skin deep, influencing how well you rest. Sleep is a cornerstone of well-being, yet many individuals struggle with poor sleep quality due to blood sugar fluctuations and imbalanced hormones. This dietary approach stabilizes blood sugar, preventing the nighttime dips that can disrupt rest. Moreover, a diet rich in protein supports the production of tryptophan, an amino acid that the body converts into serotonin and melatonin—neurotransmitters that regulate sleep cycles. As a result, you may find yourself falling asleep more easily, staying asleep longer, and waking up feeling genuinely refreshed.

Improved sleep also enhances your body's ability to recover and regenerate. The body balances hormones, fortifies the immune system, and repairs tissues as you sleep deeply. This diet's capacity to promote restorative sleep amplifies these effects, contributing to better physical health, sharper cognitive function, and even greater resilience to stress. It's a cycle of well-being that begins with your plate and reverberates through every aspect of your life.

The diet's profound influence on emotional well-being is equally remarkable. High-carb diets, with their sharp energy spikes and crashes, can wreak havoc on mental health, often triggering irritability, anxiety, and even feelings of depression. By promoting stable blood sugar levels and providing a steady, reliable energy source, this dietary approach fosters a sense of balance and emotional steadiness, creating a solid foundation for mental resilience.

Proteins in the diet are particularly important for mental health, as they supply the amino acids needed to produce dopamine and serotonin—neurotransmitters that regulate mood and motivation. These biochemical effects, combined with the psychological boost of achieving health goals, create a more positive and stable outlook.

This diet's ability to reduce inflammation plays a significant role in enhancing mental clarity and fostering emotional stability. With research increasingly linking chronic inflammation to mood disorders, it's evident that consuming processed carbs and sugars can intensify symptoms of anxiety and depression. By focusing on whole, unprocessed foods, this dietary approach naturally reduces inflammatory markers, nurtures a healthy gut microbiota, and strengthens the vital connection between the body and mind.

The overarching theme of this diet is balance—not just in macronutrient ratios, but in how it aligns your body's systems to work in harmony. From the physical to the emotional, each benefit reinforces the others, creating a positive feedback loop of wellness. Whether it's the confidence that comes from glowing skin, the vitality of a good night's sleep, or the peace of a stable mood, this diet equips you to live your best, most vibrant life.

The Star Ingredients

High-Quality Proteins: The Foundation of Optimal Nutrition

The cornerstone of the Low Carb High Protein diet lies in the thoughtful selection of high-quality proteins. These proteins are not merely a macronutrient; they are the building blocks of life, essential for supporting muscle health, enhancing metabolic function, and providing long-lasting satiety. A well-rounded approach to protein consumption includes lean meats, fresh fish, eggs, dairy products, and innovative plant-based alternatives, each contributing uniquely to a balanced and vibrant diet.

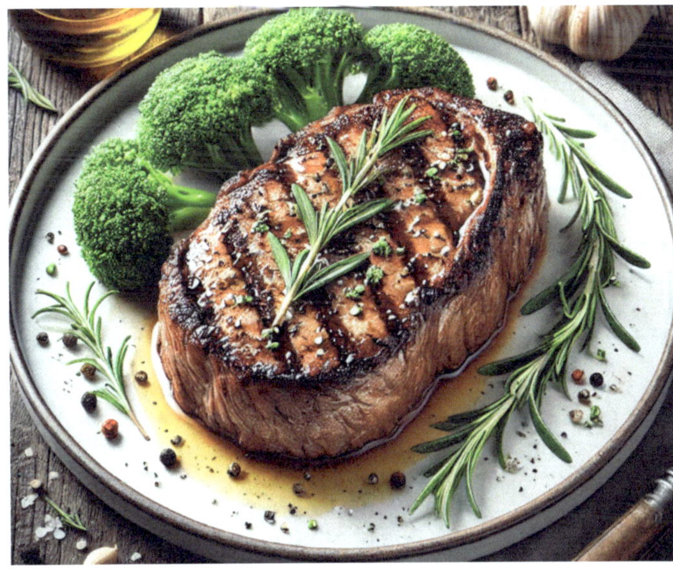

Lean meats are a classic and nutrient-rich source of protein, celebrated for their versatility and taste. Chicken, turkey, and lean cuts of beef or pork offer a concentrated dose of essential amino acids while remaining relatively low in calories and fats. These proteins are particularly beneficial for those aiming to preserve or build muscle mass, as their complete amino acid profiles ensure efficient recovery and repair of muscle tissues. Additionally, lean meats are rich in vital nutrients like iron, zinc, and B vitamins, which play critical roles in energy production and immune support.

Fish, another powerhouse of high-quality protein, brings additional health benefits that extend beyond its protein content. Fatty fish like salmon, mackerel, and sardines are abundant in omega-3 fatty acids, which are renowned for their anti-inflammatory properties and cardiovascular support. White fish, such as cod and haddock, provide leaner options that deliver protein without significant fat content, making them ideal for those focusing on caloric balance. The inclusion of fish in your diet not only supports muscle maintenance but also contributes to cognitive health, skin vitality, and overall well-being.

Eggs, often hailed as a perfect protein, deserve their reputation for versatility and nutrient density. Each egg contains a complete set of essential amino acids, along with choline—a nutrient critical for brain health and cell membrane integrity. Beyond their protein content, eggs are a source of selenium and vitamin D, nutrients that are often underrepresented in typical diets. The ability to prepare eggs in a variety of ways—from boiled to scrambled, or incorporated into savory dishes—makes them a staple in this dietary lifestyle.

Dairy products, particularly those high in protein and low in sugar, add another dimension to the diet. Greek yogurt, cottage cheese, and aged cheeses provide a creamy and satisfying way to meet daily protein needs. These options are rich in calcium and probiotics, supporting bone health and gut function. Lactose-free or reduced-fat versions are widely available for those who are sensitive to lactose or prefer to limit their fat intake. Incorporating dairy into your diet can add variety and richness while maintaining alignment with the diet's principles.

Plant-based alternatives are an increasingly popular and accessible way to diversify protein intake. For those seeking to reduce their reliance on animal products, options like tofu, tempeh, and seitan offer robust protein content with unique flavors and textures. Legumes, such as lentils and chickpeas, though slightly higher in carbohydrates, can still fit into a low-carb regimen when portioned thoughtfully. These alternatives are not only rich in protein but also supply fiber, vitamins, and minerals, contributing to overall health and digestive well-being.

Combining protein sources is a practical strategy to ensure a diverse intake of amino acids and other micronutrients. For example, pairing eggs with a side of salmon or incorporating nuts into a yogurt-based snack creates meals that are not only nutritionally complete but also deeply satisfying. This approach allows flexibility in meal planning while optimizing nutrient density.

"Good Carbohydrates": The Backbone of Nutrient Density

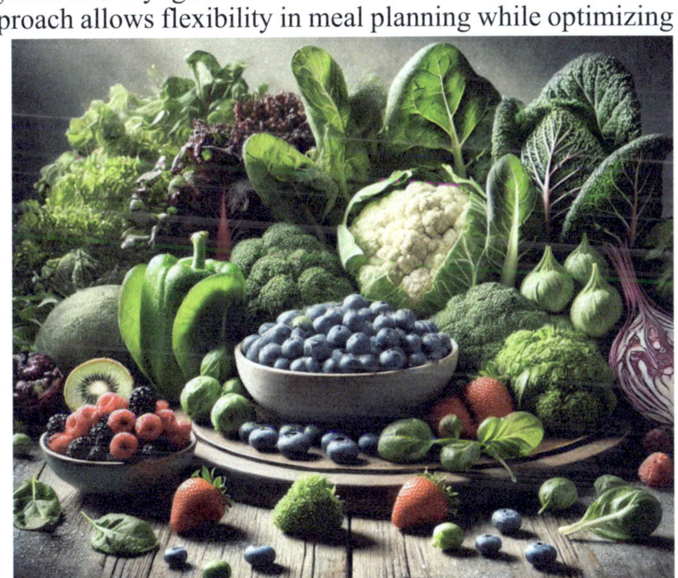

In the Low Carb High Protein diet, carbohydrates are not banished; rather, they are selected with purpose and precision. The focus is on high quality, nutrient-dense sources that provide essential vitamins, minerals, and fiber without the insulin-spiking properties of refined sugars and starches. These "good carbohydrates" include leafy greens, cruciferous vegetables, and low-glycemic fruits, which serve as nutritional powerhouses, complementing the protein-rich foundation of the diet.

Leafy greens, such as spinach, kale, and Swiss chard, are quintessential elements of a low-carb lifestyle. Rich in vitamins A, C, and K, as well as folate and iron, these vegetables provide an impressive nutrient profile with minimal carbohydrates. Their high fiber content not only supports digestive health but also contributes to feelings of satiety, making them ideal for weight management. The versatility of leafy greens allows them to shine in salads, smoothies, or sautéed dishes, seamlessly integrating into a variety of meals. Their phytonutrient content also helps reduce inflammation and oxidative stress, supporting overall cellular health.

Cruciferous vegetables, including broccoli, cauliflower, Brussels sprouts, and cabbage, are another cornerstone of good carbohydrates in the diet. These vegetables stand out for their high fiber content and unique sulfur-containing compounds, such as glucosinolates, which are known to support liver detoxification and may have anti-cancer properties. Cruciferous vegetables also provide a satisfying crunch and robust flavor, making them a versatile ingredient for everything from roasted side dishes to creamy low-carb soups. Their relatively low carbohydrate count ensures that they fit perfectly within the framework, while their dense nutrient composition enhances the diet's overall health benefits.

Low-glycemic fruits, such as berries, offer a touch of natural sweetness while maintaining compatibility with the low-carb principles of the diet. Blueberries, strawberries, raspberries, and blackberries are particularly noteworthy for their high antioxidant content, which combats free radical damage and promotes healthy aging. These fruits also contain fiber and a modest amount of natural sugars, providing a balanced energy boost without the dramatic blood sugar spikes associated with higher-glycemic fruits like bananas or pineapples. Incorporating a handful of berries into yogurt, salads, or even savory dishes adds both flavor and a wealth of health benefits to any meal.

The inclusion of good carbohydrates in the diet serves more than just nutritional purposes; it elevates the overall dining experience. These vegetables and fruits provide vibrant colors, varied textures, and a range of flavors that prevent monotony and encourage adherence to the diet over the long term. Moreover, their high water content aids in hydration, while their fiber ensures steady digestion and contributes to the feeling of fullness, reducing the likelihood of overeating.

In addition to their direct nutritional benefits, good carbohydrates play a critical role in enhancing the body's metabolic efficiency. The high fiber content in leafy greens and cruciferous vegetables slows the digestion of carbohydrates, leading to a gradual release of glucose into the bloodstream. This helps maintain stable blood sugar levels, which is essential for sustained energy and reduced cravings. Low-glycemic fruits, with their natural sugars bound to fiber, further support this balance, offering a gentle energy lift without triggering an insulin surge.

The diet transforms what might otherwise feel like a restrictive approach into an abundant and satisfying way of eating by prioritizing high-quality carbohydrate sources. These carefully selected "good carbs" not only support weight loss and muscle retention but also provide the essential nutrients needed for overall health and vitality. Although the quantity of carbohydrates is reduced, their superior quality underscores that, in the pursuit of optimal nutrition, less can indeed mean more.

Healthy Fats: Fuel for Body and Mind

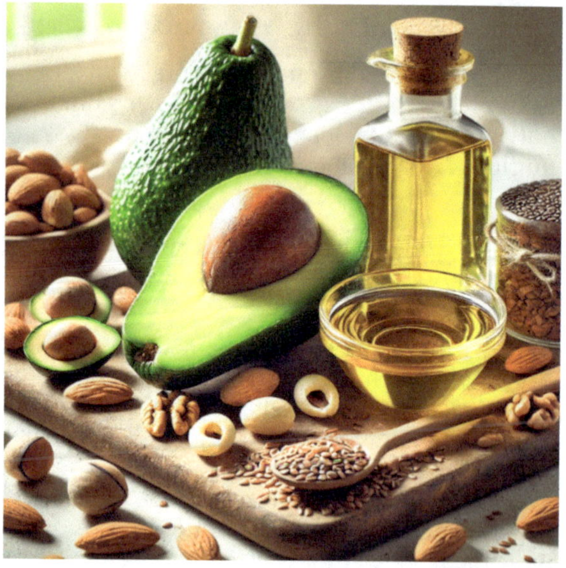

The inclusion of healthy fats in the Low Carb High Protein diet serves as a cornerstone for balanced nutrition, offering sustained energy, enhanced cellular function, and numerous health benefits. Avocado, olive oil, nuts, and seeds are exemplary sources of these fats, providing essential nutrients while complementing the protein-rich and low-carb focus of this dietary approach.

Avocado, often considered a superfood, is rich in monounsaturated fats, particularly oleic acid, which is renowned for its anti-inflammatory properties and heart health benefits. Beyond its fat profile, avocado is a powerhouse of potassium, magnesium, and fiber, nutrients that support muscle function, electrolyte balance, and digestive health. Its creamy texture and versatile flavor make it a favorite in everything from smoothies and salads to spreads and garnishes. Avocado not only enhances satiety but also supports skin elasticity and hydration, aligning with the holistic benefits of this lifestyle.

Olive oil, a staple of the Mediterranean diet, finds its rightful place in this framework as a source of high-quality fat. Extra virgin olive oil is abundant in antioxidants, such as polyphenols, which protect cells from oxidative stress and support cardiovascular health. Its anti-inflammatory effects extend to joint health and overall vitality, making it a vital addition to meals. Used as a drizzle over vegetables, a dressing base, or a cooking medium, olive oil elevates the flavor and nutritional value of dishes without adding unnecessary carbohydrates. Its role in promoting brain health and reducing the risk of chronic diseases further underscores its importance in a healthy diet.

Nuts, including almonds, walnuts, and macadamia nuts, are nutrient-dense sources of healthy fats, fiber, and protein. Almonds, for example, are rich in vitamin E and magnesium, nutrients that support immune function and energy production. Walnuts provide a unique source of plant-based omega-3 fatty acids, essential for reducing inflammation and supporting brain function. Macadamia nuts, with their buttery texture, are particularly high in monounsaturated fats, which are beneficial for heart health. Nuts offer versatility in the kitchen, serving as snacks, salad toppings, or components in low-carb baking. Their satisfying crunch and nutrient density make them indispensable in this regimen.

Seeds, such as chia, flaxseeds, and pumpkin seeds, add another layer of nutritional depth to the diet. Chia and flaxseeds are celebrated for their high fiber content and omega-3 fatty acids, which aid in digestion and support cardiovascular health. Pumpkin seeds, rich in zinc and magnesium, contribute to immune health and stress resilience. These seeds can be easily incorporated into smoothies, yogurt, or baked goods, adding texture and a nutritional boost without compromising carbohydrate goals. Their role in maintaining balanced hormones and supporting metabolic health highlights their importance in a comprehensive diet plan.

Incorporating these healthy fats achieves much more than simply fulfilling macronutrient needs; it elevates overall well-being. These fats deliver sustained energy, help maintain stable blood sugar levels, and minimize cravings, making them an essential element of a balanced lifestyle. Choosing nutrient-dense fat sources brings remarkable benefits, including sharper cognitive function, enhanced joint health, and radiant skin. This thoughtful focus on quality over quantity transforms every meal into a flavorful and nourishing experience, empowering both the body and mind to thrive.

Beverages and Seasonings: Elevating Flavor Without Compromising Goals

The Low Carb High Protein diet emphasizes not only nutrient-rich foods but also the subtle art of enhancing flavor without excess calories. Infusions, herbal teas, and spices take center stage as essential tools for creating vibrant, satisfying meals and drinks. They contribute depth and variety to the diet while aligning perfectly with its principles.

Herbal infusions and teas are more than just comforting beverages; they are functional tools in a low-carb lifestyle. Peppermint tea, for instance, aids digestion and provides a refreshing pick-me-up without any added sugar. Chamomile, known for its calming properties, supports better sleep, an essential component of overall wellness. Green tea, a powerhouse of antioxidants, can boost metabolism and aid fat oxidation, making it a valuable ally in achieving weight management goals. These beverages are naturally free of carbohydrates and calories, offering a range of options for hydration and relaxation while supporting the body's natural processes.

Spices and herbs transform simple dishes into culinary masterpieces, elevating both flavor and nutritional value. Turmeric, with its active compound curcumin, is celebrated for its anti-inflammatory properties. A pinch added to soups, stews, or scrambled eggs can not only enhance color but also deliver significant health benefits. Cinnamon, known for its ability to stabilize blood sugar levels, pairs beautifully with protein-rich yogurt or low-glycemic fruits like berries. Paprika and cayenne pepper bring a gentle heat and support circulation, adding excitement to roasted vegetables or grilled meats.

Fresh herbs like basil, cilantro, and parsley go beyond garnish status to become central components of meals. Their vibrant flavors brighten salads, marinades, and dressings without the need for sugar-laden sauces. Cilantro, in particular, offers a unique detoxifying effect, helping to rid the body of heavy metals. Basil is a rich source of vitamin K and contains compounds that support cardiovascular health, while parsley provides a dose of vitamin C and antioxidants.

Healthy beverages and condiments allow for creativity and variety, ensuring adherence to the diet's principles while keeping meals enjoyable and flavorful. These simple additions demonstrate how even the smallest details can play a significant role in a health-conscious, delicious lifestyle.

Practical Guide to Getting Started

Starting Without Stress: A Gradual and Strategic Transition

Starting the LCHP diet should inspire confidence and excitement, not leave you feeling daunted. Gradually reducing carbohydrates, combined with thoughtful meal planning, helps you transition seamlessly into this lifestyle, reducing stress and paving the way for lasting success. Taking these deliberate steps establishes a solid foundation for reaching your health and wellness goals with ease.

Gradual reduction in carbohydrate intake is essential for avoiding the common pitfalls associated with drastic dietary changes. Instead of immediately eliminating all carb-heavy foods, start by identifying and replacing the most obvious sources of refined carbohydrates, such as sugary snacks, sodas, and processed bread. Transitioning to nutrient-dense alternatives, like leafy greens and low-glycemic vegetables, helps maintain satiety and energy levels while your body adjusts to a lower carbohydrate intake. This approach not only prevents energy crashes but also allows your body to gradually adapt to using fats as its primary energy source.

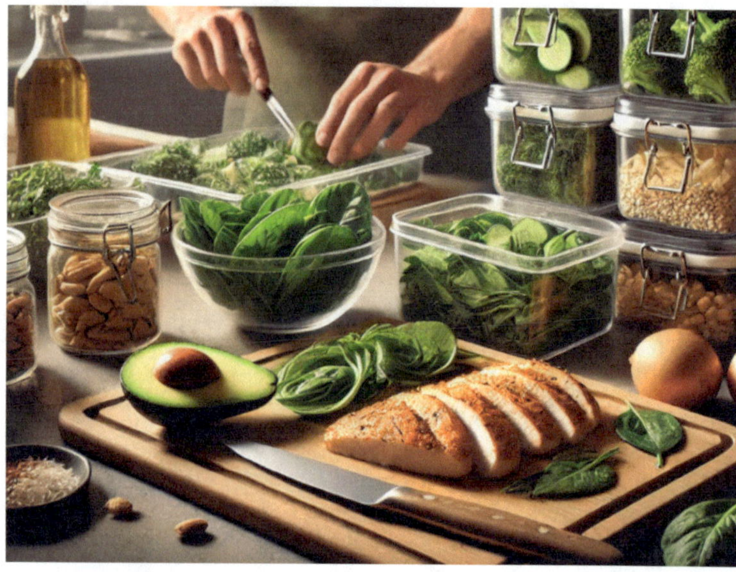

The goal is to find a rhythm that works for you. Begin by incorporating one or two low-carb meals into your daily routine, gradually increasing their frequency over a few weeks. For example, start with a high-protein breakfast featuring eggs and avocado, or a lunch with grilled chicken and a generous portion of sautéed spinach. Over time, you can phase out carb-heavy side dishes at dinner, replacing them with roasted vegetables or a fresh salad. This step-by-step process helps reduce carb cravings, stabilizes blood sugar levels, and minimizes potential side effects like fatigue or headaches that can occur when transitioning too quickly.

Organizing meals in advance serves as a fundamental pillar of this diet, seamlessly blending convenience with nutritional precision. Set aside a dedicated moment each week to craft a meal plan that incorporates a diverse array of protein sources, nutrient-rich vegetables, and wholesome fats. This thoughtful preparation streamlines your weekday routine and guarantees that each dish supports your health objectives. Aim to design well-rounded plates that deliver the muscle-sustaining power of protein, the digestive benefits of fiber, and the enduring energy provided by healthy fats.

Batch cooking is an invaluable tool for simplifying meal preparation. Prepare larger portions of proteins such as grilled chicken, roasted salmon, or marinated tofu, along with roasted vegetables like broccoli or cauliflower. Store these in individual portions that can be quickly assembled into meals throughout the week. Pairing these proteins with simple garnishes, such as a drizzle of olive oil or a handful of fresh herbs, keeps flavors exciting while requiring minimal effort.

Stocking your pantry with essentials ensures that you're always equipped to make quick and nutritious meals. Keep staples like canned tuna, nuts, seeds, and high-quality oils on hand. For vegetables, frozen options such as spinach, zucchini, or riced cauliflower are convenient and just as nutrient-packed as their fresh counterparts. These items make it easy to create satisfying meals, even when time is limited or unexpected challenges arise.

As you plan your meals, consider including small indulgences that align with this lifestyle to maintain satisfaction and reduce feelings of restriction. For example, incorporate a few dark chocolate shavings into your yogurt or enjoy a creamy dressing made from Greek yogurt and fresh herbs. These touches not only add variety but also make the diet feel more approachable and enjoyable.

During the initial transition period, tracking your meals and their effects on your energy levels can provide valuable insights. Use a journal or a food-tracking app to monitor how different meals make you feel. This practice helps identify foods that work best for your body and refine your approach over time. Pay attention to patterns, such as how high-protein breakfasts sustain you throughout the morning or how incorporating more vegetables enhances your digestion.

The shift to this diet is not only a physical journey but also a mental one. Setting realistic goals and celebrating small victories, like successfully planning a week's worth of meals or conquering carb cravings, keeps you motivated. A gradual approach and thoughtful preparation ensure that this transition is a positive, sustainable step toward long-term health and vitality.

Pantry Organization: Building the Foundation for Success

A well-organized pantry is the backbone of a successful Low Carb High Protein (LCHP) lifestyle. It allows you to make nutritious choices effortlessly, ensures you have the right ingredients on hand, and transforms meal preparation into a seamless experience. Thoughtful planning and organization of your pantry create a space that supports your health goals while eliminating the guesswork.

To simplify access to essential ingredients, consider arranging your cupboard into clearly defined sections. Dedicate one area to proteins, including canned fish such as tuna and salmon, which are quick, high-quality options for any meal. Add shelf-stable plant-based proteins like lentils or edamame to diversify your choices—while these contain carbohydrates, their high fiber content makes them valuable, occasional additions to a low-carb diet. Ensure your freezer is stocked with versatile protein staples like chicken, beef, or tofu, providing a reliable foundation for effortless meal preparation.

Next, focus on building a robust collection of nutrient-dense, low-carb vegetables. While these are typically stored fresh, having frozen options like spinach, broccoli, and riced cauliflower ensures you're never without a quick, healthy base for meals. These frozen staples maintain their nutritional integrity and eliminate concerns about spoilage, making them indispensable for busy schedules.

Include a section for healthy fats, which are essential for this diet. Organize bottles of high-quality oils, such as olive, avocado, and coconut oil, in a cool, dark area to preserve their freshness. Keep nuts and seeds, such as almonds, walnuts, chia, and flaxseeds, in airtight containers to maintain their crunch and nutritional value. In addition to adding taste, these fats supply vital fatty acids that promote fullness and energy.

Spices and condiments are another critical component of your pantry. A well-curated spice collection, including turmeric, paprika, and cinnamon, ensures your meals remain flavorful and diverse without adding unnecessary calories or sugars. Low-carb condiments such as mustard, apple cider vinegar, and sugar-free hot sauces add zest to your dishes while aligning with dietary goals. For dressings and marinades, stock up on items like tahini or Greek yogurt, which can be paired with fresh herbs for homemade, health-conscious creations.

Investing in high-quality storage solutions can elevate your pantry organization and make meal preparation more efficient. Use transparent, labeled containers for dry goods like nuts, seeds, and protein powders, allowing you to quickly identify what's available. Organize shelves by frequency of use, placing everyday items like oils and spices within easy reach, while reserving higher shelves for bulk or backup ingredients.

Efficient pantry organization also includes preparing for unexpected moments when time or motivation is scarce. Assemble a few ready-to-go meal kits with all the necessary components for a quick, balanced meal. For instance, combine canned tuna, a small packet of olive oil, and pre-portioned nuts for an emergency lunch option. Similarly, frozen protein, riced vegetables, and a jar of marinara sauce can create a satisfying dinner with minimal effort.

Planning your grocery shopping around pantry essentials helps maintain an organized space while avoiding unnecessary purchases. Start with a checklist of staple items and replenish only what is running low. This strategy minimizes clutter and ensures your pantry remains a streamlined, functional resource for your dietary journey. Prioritizing quality over quantity is key—investing in fresh, nutrient-dense foods eliminates the temptation of processed or non-compliant items.

Creating a well-stocked, carefully organized pantry goes beyond mere practicality; it becomes a powerful statement of commitment. By filling your space with nourishing foods and clearing away barriers to healthy choices, you craft an environment that naturally supports your dedication. This solid foundation streamlines your daily routine and gives you the confidence and ease to pursue your health goals effectively.

Strategies for Success: Navigating the First Weeks and Staying Motivated

The first few weeks of embracing the lifestyle are pivotal in shaping your journey toward lasting success. By approaching this transition with thoughtful strategies, you can navigate challenges, establish sustainable habits, and maintain your enthusiasm. This period is not just about altering what you eat—it's an opportunity to transform how you connect with food and prioritize your overall well-being.

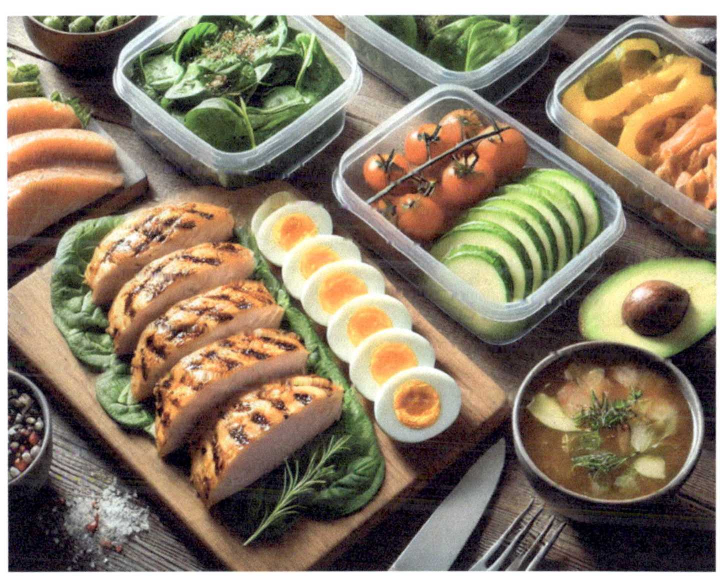

The initial weeks of transitioning to a low-carb diet mark an important adjustment period for your body. As you reduce carbohydrate intake, your system shifts to using fats as its primary energy source—a natural process that can sometimes trigger temporary effects like fatigue or irritability. To minimize these challenges, focus on staying well-hydrated and ensuring your diet includes plenty of electrolytes. Foods rich in potassium, magnesium, and sodium—such as spinach, avocado, and bone broth—play a crucial role in maintaining energy levels and supporting your body during this adaptation.

Focus on consistency rather than perfection. The goal is to gradually build a routine that aligns with your lifestyle and preferences. Begin with simple, manageable changes, such as replacing one high-carb meal with a low-carb alternative or swapping sugary snacks for high-protein options like Greek yogurt or a handful of nuts. Each small adjustment brings you closer to making the approach second nature.

Meal preparation is a cornerstone of success in this diet. Planning and preparing meals ahead of time not only saves effort during busy days but also reduces the temptation to reach for non-compliant foods. Set aside a few hours each week to cook proteins like chicken breasts, boiled eggs, or grilled fish, and pair them with pre-chopped vegetables or low-glycemic fruits. Keep these in separate pieces so you can easily reach them all week long. A well-stocked pantry and freezer ensure that even on your busiest days, you can create nourishing, satisfying meals in minutes.

Tracking your progress is another powerful tool for staying motivated. Use a journal or app to record not only your meals but also how you feel physically and mentally. Noticing patterns, such as improved energy after high-protein breakfasts or reduced cravings after incorporating healthy fats, reinforces the benefits of the diet and encourages adherence. Celebrate milestones, no matter how small—whether it's consistently planning meals for a week or feeling less reliant on sugary snacks.

The secret to overcome possible obstacles is creating a supportive environment. Share your goals with friends or family members and invite them to join you in preparing or enjoying friendly meals. Online communities and forums can also provide encouragement, recipe ideas, and insights from others on the same journey. Surrounding yourself with a network of like-minded individuals helps maintain enthusiasm and accountability.

Flexibility is another critical component of long-term success. Life is unpredictable, and there will be moments when sticking rigidly to the plan feels challenging. Approach these situations with a mindset of balance rather than restriction. For example, if you're dining out, focus on ordering dishes that emphasize proteins and vegetables while skipping the bread or dessert. If you do indulge, view it as a momentary detour rather than a failure, and simply return to your routine at the next meal.

Mindset plays a pivotal role in sustaining motivation. Shift your focus from what you're avoiding to what you're gaining—improved energy, mental clarity, and overall well-being. Visualize your goals and remind yourself why you started. Create a list of positive affirmations or motivational quotes to revisit whenever you need a boost. This mental resilience is just as important as the physical changes you're pursuing.

Remember that this diet is more than a short-term solution; it's a lifestyle designed to support lasting health and vitality. Embracing a thoughtful approach grounded in preparation, steady adjustments, and a positive mindset creates the foundation for long-term success. Above all, your commitment to prioritizing your well-being becomes the most powerful driving force behind this transformative journey.

Reference Tables for a Low Carb High Protein Diet

A well-structured diet starts with clear reference points, particularly when distinguishing between low-carb and high-protein foods. This section categorizes key ingredients, providing guidance for meal planning and nutrient tracking. Additionally, an overview of macronutrient calculations ensures you can tailor the diet to your specific needs.

Categorization of Foods

Below is a breakdown of foods suitable for a Low Carb High Protein diet, grouped by their primary macronutrient contribution. These foods are nutrient-dense, minimally processed, and optimized for satiety and metabolic efficiency.

Calculating Macronutrients

Tracking macronutrients ensures that your diet aligns with your health goals. Here's how to calculate your daily macronutrient needs and distribute them effectively within the LCHP framework:

How to Calculate Your Total Caloric Needs

1. **Determine Your Basal Metabolic Rate (BMR):** Use the following formulas to calculate your BMR, which represents the number of calories your body burns at rest.
    - **For Women:** BMR = (10 × weight in kg) + (6.25 × height in cm) − (5 × age) − 161
    - **For Men:** BMR = (10 × weight in kg) + (6.25 × height in cm) − (5 × age) + 5
2. **Adjust for Activity Level:** Multiply your BMR by an activity factor based on your lifestyle to determine your total daily caloric needs:
    - Sedentary (little to no exercise): **BMR × 1.2**
    - Light activity (light exercise/sports 1–3 days/week): **BMR × 1.375**
    - Moderate activity (moderate exercise/sports 3–5 days/week): **BMR × 1.55**
    - Very active (hard exercise/sports 6–7 days/week): **BMR × 1.725**
    - Extra active (very hard exercise/physical job): **BMR × 1.9**

This calculation gives you the total calories your body needs daily to maintain its current weight based on your activity level. Adjust caloric intake according to your specific goals, such as weight loss or muscle gain.

1. **Set Macronutrient Ratios** The LCHP diet typically adheres to these macronutrient percentages:
    - **Protein**: 30-40%
    - **Carbohydrates**: 10-20%
    - **Fats**: 40-50%
2. For example, a 2,000-calorie daily intake would allocate:
    - Protein: 600-800 kcal (150-200g)
    - Carbohydrates: 200-400 kcal (50-100g)
    - Fats: 800-1,000 kcal (89-111g)
3. **Customize Based on Goals**
    - **Weight Loss**: Reduce total calorie intake by 10-20%.
    - **Muscle Gain**: Increase protein intake to 1.6-2.2 grams per kilogram of body weight.
    - **Maintenance**: Focus on maintaining balanced macronutrient ratios.

Category	Food Examples	Notes
Proteins	Chicken breast, turkey, lean beef, pork tenderloin, eggs, tofu, seitan, tempeh	Emphasize lean cuts and plant-based alternatives for variety.
Fish & Seafood	Salmon, tuna, mackerel, cod, shrimp, scallops	Fatty fish like salmon provide omega-3s; lean fish like cod are high in protein.
Low-Carb Veggies	Spinach, kale, zucchini, broccoli, cauliflower, asparagus, bell peppers	Rich in fiber and essential vitamins; ideal for meal bases or side dishes.
Fruits	Strawberries, blueberries, raspberries, blackberries	Stick to berries due to their low glycemic index and high antioxidant content.
Healthy Fats	Avocado, olive oil, coconut oil, almonds, walnuts, chia seeds, flaxseeds	Use as dressing, cooking oil, or snacks to meet fat requirements while keeping carbs low.
Dairy	Greek yogurt (unsweetened), cottage cheese, aged cheese (cheddar, Parmesan)	Focus on low-lactose options to minimize carbohydrates.
Condiments & Spices	Mustard, apple cider vinegar, turmeric, paprika, chili flakes	Enhance flavors without adding hidden sugars or excessive calories.

Example Daily Plan

Meal	Ingredients	Macronutrient Breakdown
Breakfast	3 eggs scrambled with spinach and a side of avocado	Protein: 20g, Carbs: 5g, Fats: 25g
Snack	1 cup Greek yogurt with 50g raspberries	Protein: 15g, Carbs: 10g, Fats: 5g
Lunch	Grilled chicken breast with zucchini noodles and olive oil drizzle	Protein: 35g, Carbs: 10g, Fats: 20g
Snack	20g almonds	Protein: 5g, Carbs: 2g, Fats: 14g
Dinner	Baked salmon with roasted cauliflower and a sprinkle of flaxseeds	Protein: 40g, Carbs: 8g, Fats: 30g

Adopting a structured approach with reference tables and precise calculations ensures that your LCHP diet remains both practical and effective, helping you achieve optimal results while enjoying every meal.

Fuel Your Body

Breakfast

Scrambled Eggs with Spinach and Feta

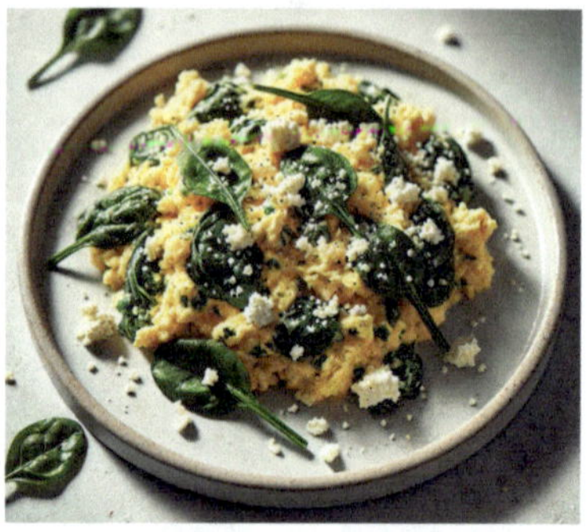

Number of servings: 2
Preparation time: 5 minutes
Cooking time: 5 minutes

Ingredients:

- 4 large eggs
- 1 cup fresh spinach, chopped
- 1/3 cup feta cheese, crumbled
- 1 tbsp olive oil or butter
- Sea salt and black pepper to taste

Directions:

1. Heat the olive oil or butter in a non-stick skillet over medium heat.
2. Add the spinach and sauté for 1-2 minutes until wilted.
3. In a bowl, whisk the eggs with a pinch of salt and pepper.
4. Pour the eggs into the skillet and cook gently, stirring occasionally, until softly scrambled.
5. Fold in the crumbled feta cheese and cook for another 1 minute until melted and incorporated.
6. Serve immediately and enjoy.

Nutritional value per serving: Calories: 210, Carbs: 2g, Fiber: 1g, Sugars: 1g, Protein: 12g, Saturated fat: 6g, Unsaturated fat: 7g

Difficulty rating: ★☆☆☆☆

Tips for ingredient variations: Add cherry tomatoes or diced bell peppers for extra flavor and nutrition. You can also substitute feta with goat cheese.

Greek Yogurt with Chia Seeds and Berries

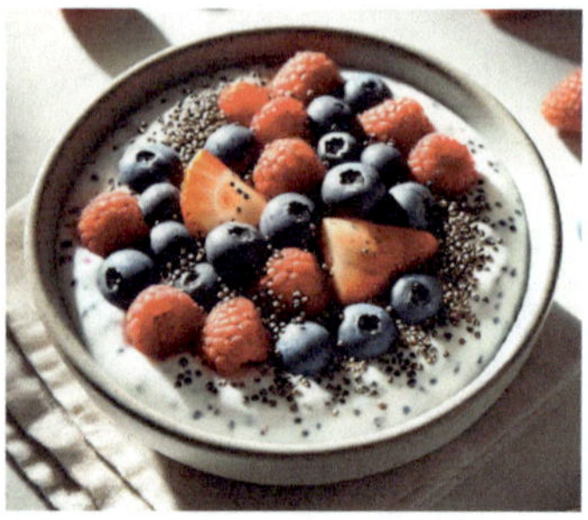

Number of servings: 1
Preparation time: 5 minutes
Cooking time: 0 minutes

Ingredients:

- 1 cup unsweetened Greek yogurt
- 1 tbsp chia seeds
- 1/4 cup mixed berries (blueberries, raspberries, or strawberries)
- 1 tsp honey or low-carb sweetener (optional)

Directions:

1. In a serving bowl, combine Greek yogurt and chia seeds. Mix well.
2. Let the mixture sit for 2-3 minutes to allow the chia seeds to soften slightly.
3. Top with mixed berries and drizzle with honey or sweetener if desired.
4. Serve immediately.

Nutritional value per serving: Calories: 160, Carbs: 9g, Fiber: 3g, Sugars: 6g, Protein: 12g, Saturated fat: 2g, Unsaturated fat: 1g

Difficulty rating: ★☆☆☆☆

Tips for ingredient variations: Sprinkle with crushed nuts like almonds or walnuts for added crunch and protein.

Avocado and Smoked Salmon Toast (on Low-Carb Bread)

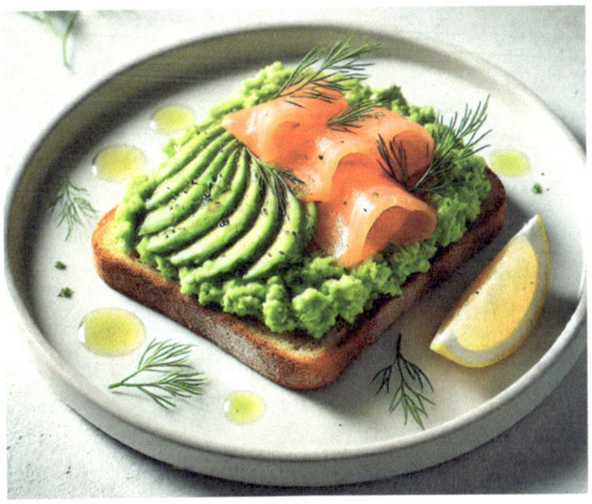

Number of servings: 1

Preparation time: 5 minutes

Cooking time: 0 minutes

Ingredients:

- 1 slice of low-carb bread, toasted
- 1/2 avocado, mashed
- 2 slices smoked salmon
- 1 tsp lemon juice
- 1 tbsp cream cheese (optional)
- Fresh dill or chives for garnish
- Sea salt and black pepper to taste

Directions:

1. Spread the mashed avocado over the toasted low-carb bread.
2. Layer the smoked salmon slices on top.
3. Drizzle with lemon juice and sprinkle with salt and pepper.
4. Garnish with fresh dill or chives. Add cream cheese as an optional layer.
5. Serve immediately.

Nutritional value per serving: Calories: 210, Carbs: 6g, Fiber: 4g, Sugars: 1g, Protein: 12g, Saturated fat: 4g, Unsaturated fat: 10g

Difficulty rating: ★☆☆☆☆

Tips for ingredient variations: Top with a poached egg for an added protein boost.

Mushroom and Cheese Omelette

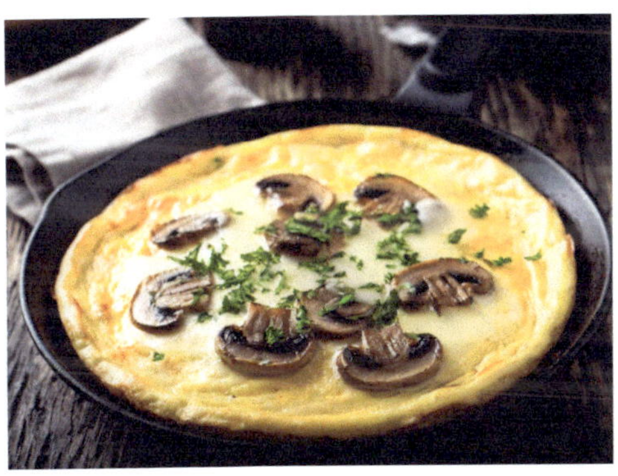

Number of servings: 1

Preparation time: 5 minutes

Cooking time: 5 minutes

Ingredients:

- 2 large eggs
- 1/2 cup mushrooms, sliced
- 1/4 cup shredded cheese (cheddar, mozzarella, or Gruyère)
- 1 tbsp butter or olive oil
- Sea salt and black pepper to taste

Directions:

1. Heat the butter or olive oil in a non-stick skillet over medium heat.
2. Add the sliced mushrooms and sauté for 2-3 minutes until softened.
3. In a bowl, whisk the eggs with a pinch of salt and pepper.
4. Pour the eggs into the skillet over the mushrooms and let cook undisturbed for 1-2 minutes.
5. Sprinkle the shredded cheese over half of the omelette.
6. Fold the omelette in half and cook for another minute until the cheese melts.
7. Slide onto a plate and serve.

Nutritional value per serving: Calories: 230, Carbs: 3g, Fiber: 1g, Sugars: 1g, Protein: 15g, Saturated fat: 7g, Unsaturated fat: 8g

Difficulty rating: ★☆☆☆☆

Tips for ingredient variations: Add spinach or diced tomatoes for extra flavor and nutrients.

Protein Pancakes (Made with Almond Flour)

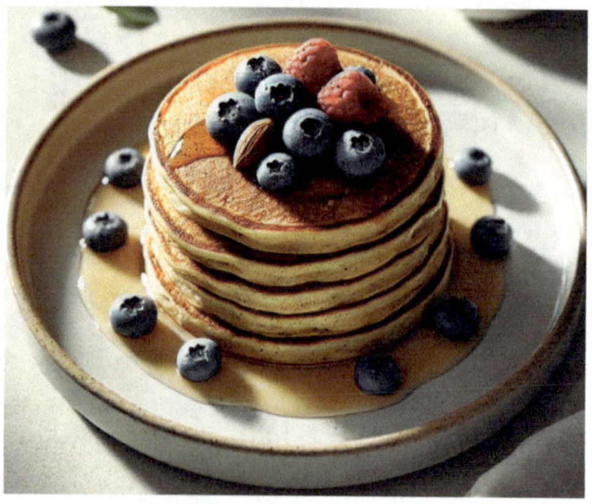

Number of servings: 2

Preparation time: 10 minutes

Cooking time: 10 minutes

Ingredients:

- 1 cup almond flour
- 2 large eggs
- 1/4 cup unsweetened almond milk
- 1 tsp vanilla extract
- 1 tsp baking powder
- 1 tsp cinnamon (optional)
- Coconut oil or butter for cooking

Directions:

1. In a bowl, mix almond flour, baking powder, and cinnamon.
2. In a separate bowl, whisk together eggs, almond milk, and vanilla extract.
3. Mix the dry ingredients with the wet ingredients gradually until they are smooth.
4. Heat a non-stick skillet over medium heat and add a small amount of coconut oil or butter.
5. Pour 2-3 tablespoons of batter for each pancake and cook for 2-3 minutes on each side until golden brown.
6. Serve warm with sugar-free syrup or a handful of fresh berries.

Nutritional value per serving: Calories: 180, Carbs: 5g, Fiber: 2g, Sugars: 1g, Protein: 10g, Saturated fat: 3g, Unsaturated fat: 7g

Difficulty rating: ★★☆☆☆

Tips for ingredient variations: Add a scoop of protein powder to the batter for an extra protein boost.

Hard-Boiled Eggs with Avocado Slices

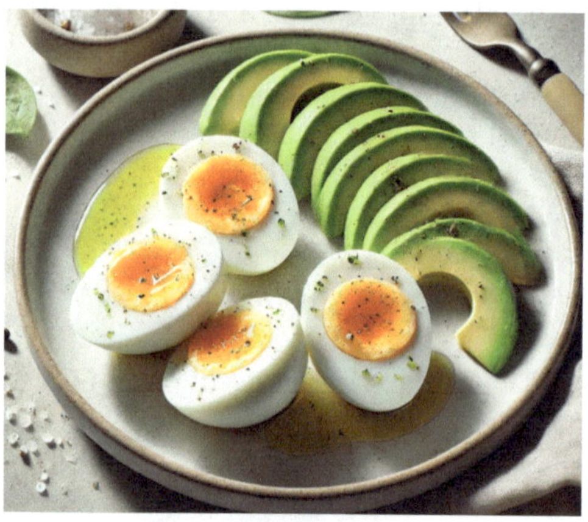

Number of servings: 1

Preparation time: 5 minutes

Cooking time: 10 minutes

Ingredients:

- 2 large eggs
- 1/2 avocado, sliced
- 1 tsp olive oil (optional)
- Sea salt and black pepper to taste

Directions:

1. Place the eggs in a saucepan and cover with water. Bring to a boil over medium-high heat.
2. Once boiling, reduce heat to low and let the eggs simmer for 9-10 minutes.
3. Remove the eggs and place them in cold water for 2-3 minutes to cool.
4. Peel the eggs and slice them in half. Arrange on a plate with the avocado slices.
5. Drizzle with olive oil if desired and sprinkle with sea salt and black pepper. Serve immediately.

Nutritional value per serving: Calories: 230, Carbs: 6g, Fiber: 4g, Sugars: 1g, Protein: 12g, Saturated fat: 3g, Unsaturated fat: 8g

Difficulty rating: ★☆☆☆☆

Tips for ingredient variations: Add a sprinkle of red pepper flakes or a drizzle of lemon juice for extra flavor.

Cottage Cheese with Cucumber and Cherry Tomatoes

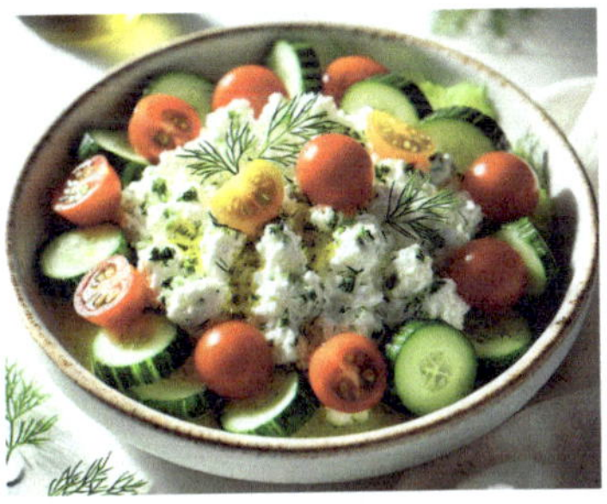

Number of servings: 1
Preparation time: 5 minutes
Cooking time: 0 minutes

Ingredients:

- 1 cup low-fat cottage cheese
- 1/4 cucumber, diced
- 5 cherry tomatoes, halved
- 1 tsp olive oil
- 1 tsp fresh dill, chopped (optional)
- Sea salt and black pepper to taste

Directions:

1. Place the cottage cheese in a serving bowl.
2. Top with diced cucumber and halved cherry tomatoes.
3. Drizzle with olive oil and season with sea salt and black pepper.
4. Garnish with fresh dill if desired and serve immediately.

Nutritional value per serving: Calories: 180, Carbs: 7g, Fiber: 1g, Sugars: 5g, Protein: 14g, Saturated fat: 2g, Unsaturated fat: 3g

Difficulty rating: ★☆☆☆☆

Tips for ingredient variations: Add a handful of arugula or a few olives for a Mediterranean twist.

Low-Carb Breakfast Burrito (with Egg Wrap)

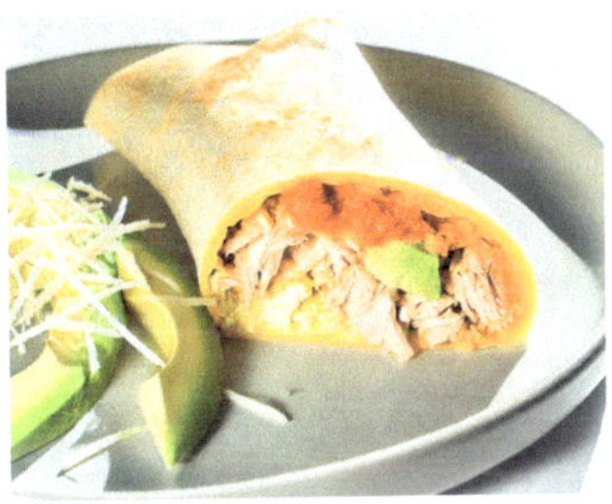

Number of servings: 1
Preparation time: 10 minutes
Cooking time: 5 minutes

Ingredients:

- 2 large eggs
- 1 tbsp heavy cream
- 1/4 cup cooked chicken or turkey, shredded
- 1/4 avocado, sliced
- 1 tbsp shredded cheese (cheddar or mozzarella)
- 1 tbsp salsa (optional)
- 1 tsp butter or olive oil

Directions:

1. Whisk the eggs and heavy cream in a bowl until combined.
2. Heat the butter or olive oil in a non-stick skillet over medium heat.
3. Pour the egg mixture into the skillet, tilting to form a thin, even layer. Cook for 2-3 minutes until set.
4. Carefully remove the egg wrap and place it on a plate.
5. Add shredded chicken or turkey, avocado slices, shredded cheese, and salsa (if using) to the center of the wrap.
6. Roll the egg wrap tightly, slice in half, and serve.

Nutritional value per serving: Calories: 280, Carbs: 3g, Fiber: 1g, Sugars: 1g, Protein: 20g, Saturated fat: 7g, Unsaturated fat: 10g

Difficulty rating: ★★☆☆☆

Tips for ingredient variations: Substitute chicken with smoked salmon or tofu for a different protein source.

Sausage and Egg Breakfast Bowl

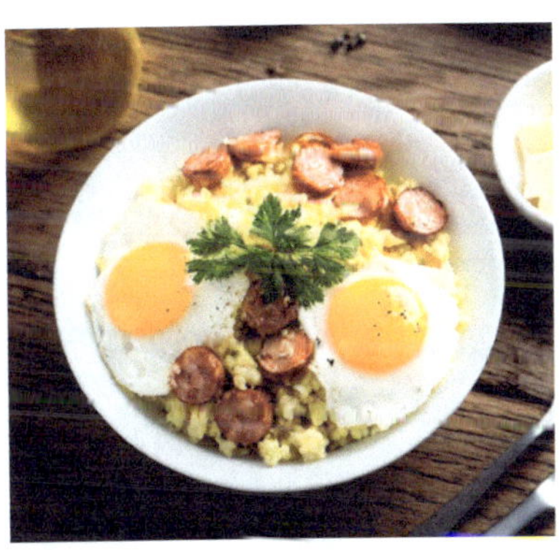

Number of servings: 1
Preparation time: 5 minutes
Cooking time: 10 minutes

Ingredients:

- 2 large eggs
- 1/4 cup breakfast sausage (crumbled, cooked)
- 1/4 cup shredded cheese (cheddar or mozzarella)
- 1/4 avocado, diced
- 1 tbsp olive oil or butter
- Sea salt and black pepper to taste

Directions:

1. Heat the olive oil or butter in a skillet over medium heat.
2. Crack the eggs into the skillet and scramble gently until cooked through.
3. Add the cooked sausage and stir to combine.
4. Transfer to a bowl and top with shredded cheese and diced avocado.
5. Season with salt and pepper and serve warm.

Nutritional value per serving: Calories: 320, Carbs: 2g, Fiber: 1g, Sugars: 0g, Protein: 21g, Saturated fat: 8g, Unsaturated fat: 12g

Difficulty rating: ★☆☆☆☆

Tips for ingredient variations: Add sautéed spinach or mushrooms for extra nutrients.

Zucchini Noodles with Fried Egg and Parmesan

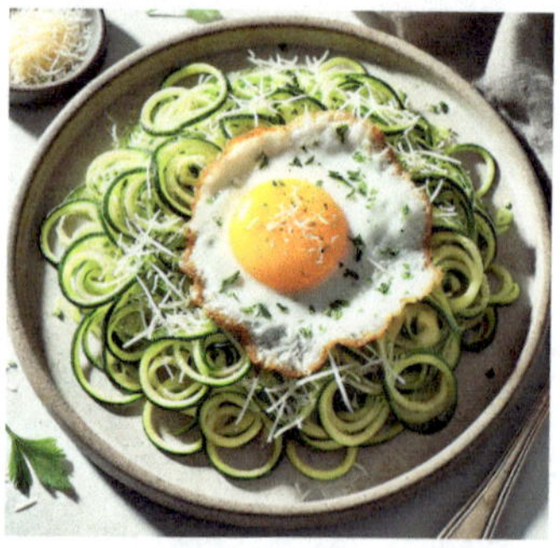

Number of servings: 2
Preparation time: 10 minutes
Cooking time: 10 minutes

Ingredients:

- 2 medium zucchinis, spiralized into noodles
- 2 large eggs
- 1/4 cup grated Parmesan cheese
- 1 tbsp olive oil
- 1 garlic clove, minced
- 1 tbsp fresh parsley, chopped (optional)
- Sea salt and black pepper to taste

Directions:

1. Heat olive oil in a skillet over medium heat. Add the minced garlic and sauté for 1-2 minutes until fragrant.
2. Add the zucchini noodles to the skillet and cook for 3-4 minutes until just tender. Season with salt and pepper.
3. In a separate skillet, fry the eggs to your desired doneness (sunny-side-up or over-easy).
4. Divide the zucchini noodles between two plates, top each with a fried egg, and sprinkle with Parmesan cheese.
5. Garnish with fresh parsley if desired and serve immediately.

Nutritional value per serving: Calories: 180, Carbs: 5g, Fiber: 2g, Sugars: 3g, Protein: 10g, Saturated fat: 4g, Unsaturated fat: 8g

Difficulty rating: ★★☆☆☆

Tips for ingredient variations: Add a pinch of chili flakes for spice or a handful of cherry tomatoes for a pop of color.

Almond Butter Smoothie with Unsweetened Almond Milk

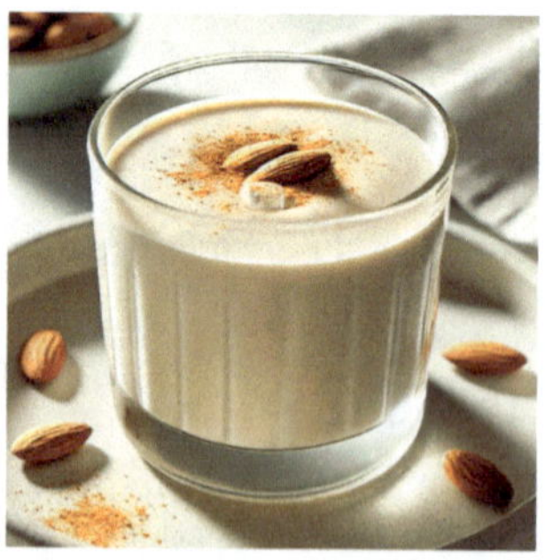

Number of servings: 1
Preparation time: 5 minutes
Cooking time: 0 minutes

Ingredients:

- 1 cup unsweetened almond milk
- 2 tbsp almond butter
- 1 scoop vanilla protein powder (low-carb)
- 1/4 tsp cinnamon
- 4-5 ice cubes
- Optional: 1 tsp chia seeds for added texture

Directions:

1. Combine almond milk, almond butter, protein powder, cinnamon, and ice cubes in a blender.
2. Blend on high until smooth and creamy.
3. Pour into a glass and serve immediately.

Nutritional value per serving: Calories: 220, Carbs: 7g, Fiber: 3g, Sugars: 1g, Protein: 20g, Saturated fat: 1g, Unsaturated fat: 8g

Difficulty rating: ★☆☆☆☆

Tips for ingredient variations: Substitute almond butter with peanut butter or add a handful of spinach for extra nutrients without altering the flavor.

Chia Pudding with Vanilla and Coconut Milk

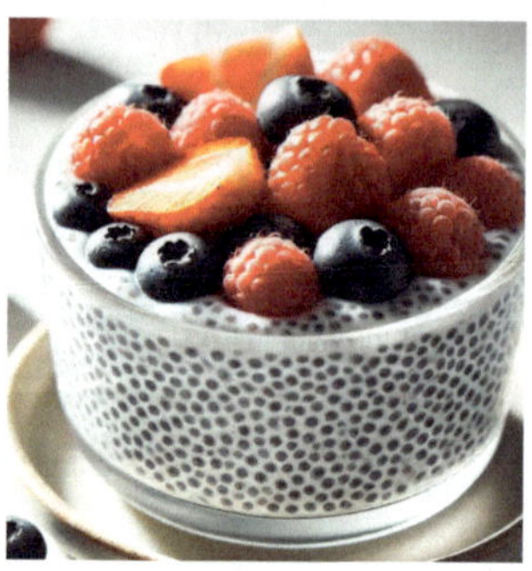

Number of servings: 2
Preparation time: 5 minutes
Cooking time: 0 minutes (refrigeration time: 4 hours or overnight)

Ingredients:

- 1 cup unsweetened coconut milk
- 3 tbsp chia seeds
- 1 tsp vanilla extract
- 1 tsp low-carb sweetener (optional)
- Fresh berries for topping

Directions:

1. In a bowl or jar, mix the coconut milk, chia seeds, vanilla extract, and sweetener until well combined.
2. Cover and refrigerate for at least 4 hours or overnight to allow the chia seeds to expand and thicken.
3. Stir the pudding before serving and top with fresh berries.

Nutritional value per serving: Calories: 180, Carbs: 6g, Fiber: 4g, Sugars: 1g, Protein: 4g, Saturated fat: 10g, Unsaturated fat: 1g

Difficulty rating: ★☆☆☆☆

Tips for ingredient variations: Add unsweetened cocoa powder for a chocolate flavor or top with chopped nuts for added crunch.

Turkey Bacon and Egg Cups

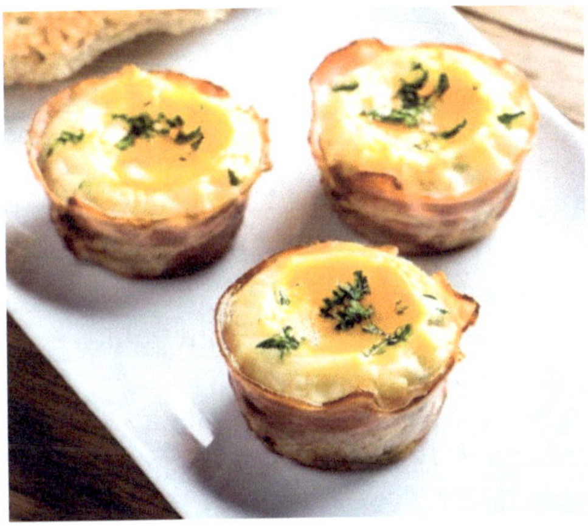

Number of servings: 6 cups (2-3 servings)

Preparation time: 10 minutes

Cooking time: 20 minutes

Ingredients:

- 6 slices turkey bacon
- 6 large eggs
- 1/4 cup shredded cheddar cheese
- 1/4 tsp black pepper
- Cooking spray

Directions:

1. Preheat the oven to 375°F (190°C) and spray a muffin tin with cooking spray.
2. Line each muffin cup with a slice of turkey bacon, forming a circle.
3. In each cup, crack one egg and season with black pepper and grated cheese.
4. The egg whites should be set after 18 to 20 minutes of baking, but the yolks should still be slightly liquid.
5. Let cool for 2 minutes before carefully removing the cups from the tin.

Nutritional value per serving (2 cups): Calories: 160, Carbs: 1g, Fiber: 0g, Sugars: 0g, Protein: 18g, Saturated fat: 4g, Unsaturated fat: 3g

Difficulty rating: ★☆☆☆☆

Tips for ingredient variations: Add chopped spinach or diced bell peppers to the cups for extra flavor and nutrition.

Low-Carb Granola with Greek Yogurt

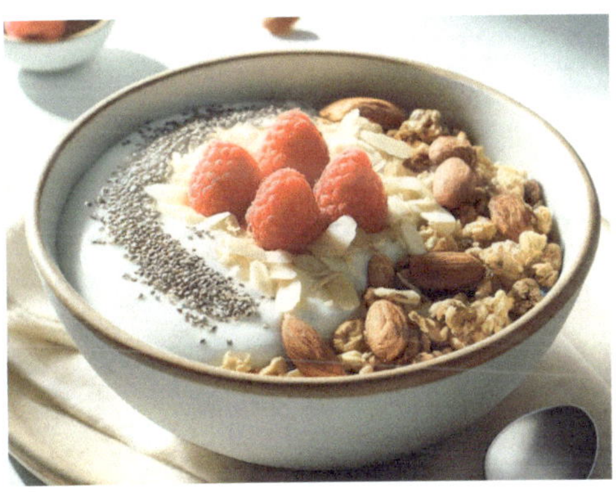

Number of servings: 1

Preparation time: 5 minutes

Cooking time: 0 minutes

Ingredients:

- 1/2 cup unsweetened Greek yogurt
- 1/4 cup low-carb granola (made with nuts and seeds)
- 1 tbsp shredded unsweetened coconut
- 1 tsp chia seeds
- Optional: a few fresh raspberries for garnish

Directions:

1. Spoon Greek yogurt into a serving bowl.
2. Top with low-carb granola, shredded coconut, and chia seeds.
3. Add fresh raspberries for garnish if desired, and serve immediately.

Nutritional value per serving: Calories: 200, Carbs: 7g, Fiber: 3g, Sugars: 2g, Protein: 15g, Saturated fat: 3g, Unsaturated fat: 5g

Difficulty rating: ★☆☆☆☆

Tips for ingredient variations: Use almond butter drizzle instead of berries for a richer taste or add cinnamon for extra warmth.

Cauliflower Hash Browns with Poached Eggs

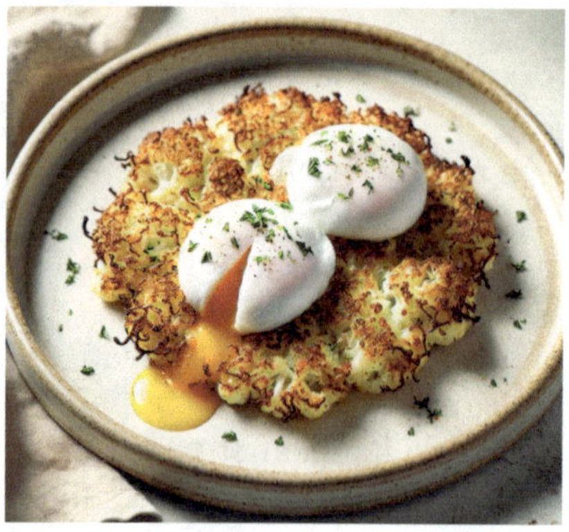

Number of servings: 2

Preparation time: 10 minutes

Cooking time: 15 minutes

Ingredients:

- 2 cups riced cauliflower
- 1/4 cup shredded Parmesan cheese
- 1 egg (for the hash browns)
- 2 large eggs (for poaching)
- 1/4 tsp garlic powder
- 1/4 tsp onion powder
- 2 tbsp olive oil or butter
- Sea salt and black pepper to taste

Directions:

1. In a bowl, mix riced cauliflower, Parmesan, one egg, garlic powder, onion powder, salt, and pepper until well combined.
2. Heat olive oil in a skillet over medium heat. Scoop small portions of the cauliflower mixture and flatten into patties.
3. Cook for 3-4 minutes per side until golden brown, then transfer to a plate.
4. In the meantime, crack one egg into a small bowl and carefully slip it into a kettle of simmering water. Poach each egg for 3-4 minutes.
5. Serve the poached eggs on top of the hash browns and enjoy warm.

Nutritional value per serving: Calories: 220, Carbs: 6g, Fiber: 2g, Sugars: 1g, Protein: 12g, Saturated fat: 3g, Unsaturated fat: 7g

Difficulty rating: ★★☆☆☆

Tips for ingredient variations: Add chopped herbs like parsley or dill to the cauliflower mixture for extra flavor.

Bell Pepper and Cheese Mini Frittatas

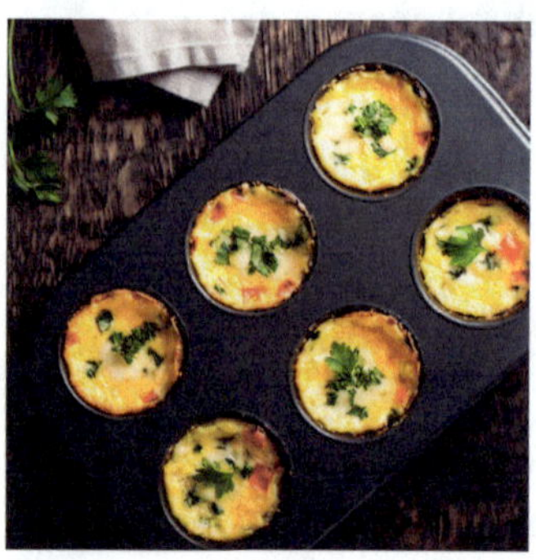

Number of servings: 4

Preparation time: 10 minutes

Cooking time: 20 minutes

Ingredients:

- 6 large eggs
- 1 cup bell peppers, diced (red, yellow, or green)
- 1/2 cup shredded cheddar or mozzarella cheese
- 1/4 cup chopped fresh parsley or chives
- 1/4 tsp salt
- 1/4 tsp black pepper
- Olive oil or cooking spray for greasing

Directions:

1. Heat the oven to 375°F (190°C) and use cooking spray or olive oil to gently coat a muffin tin.
2. In a mixing bowl, whisk together the eggs, salt, and black pepper until well combined.
3. Fold in the diced bell peppers, shredded cheese, and parsley or chives.
4. Pour the mixture evenly into the muffin tin, filling each cup about 3/4 full.
5. Bake for 18-20 minutes or until the frittatas are set and slightly golden on top.
6. Let cool for a few minutes before serving.

Nutritional value per serving: Calories: 120, Carbs: 3g, Fiber: 1g, Sugars: 1g, Protein: 8g, Saturated fat: 3g, Unsaturated fat: 4g

Difficulty rating: ★☆☆☆☆

Tips for ingredient variations: Add cooked bacon or diced mushrooms for additional flavor. These frittatas can also be refrigerated for a quick grab-and-go breakfast.

Keto Waffles (Almond Flour and Cream Cheese-Based)

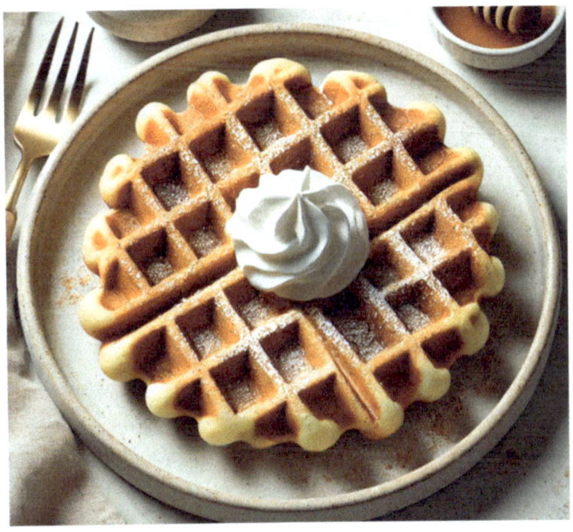

Number of servings: 2

Preparation time: 10 minutes

Cooking time: 10 minutes

Ingredients:

- 1/2 cup almond flour
- 2 large eggs
- 2 tbsp cream cheese, softened
- 1/4 tsp baking powder
- 1/4 tsp vanilla extract
- Butter or coconut oil for greasing

Directions:

1. Preheat a waffle iron and grease lightly with butter or coconut oil.
2. In a mixing bowl, whisk together almond flour, baking powder, eggs, cream cheese, and vanilla extract until smooth.
3. After the waffle iron has been preheated, pour the batter into it and cook it for the recommended amount of time, usually three to five minutes, or until golden brown.
4. Serve warm with sugar-free syrup or a dollop of whipped cream.

Nutritional value per serving: Calories: 210, Carbs: 4g, Fiber: 1g, Sugars: 1g, Protein: 10g, Saturated fat: 7g, Unsaturated fat: 5g

Difficulty rating: ★★☆☆☆

Tips for ingredient variations: Add a sprinkle of cinnamon or a handful of sugar-free chocolate chips to the batter for extra flavor.

Spinach and Ricotta Breakfast Bake

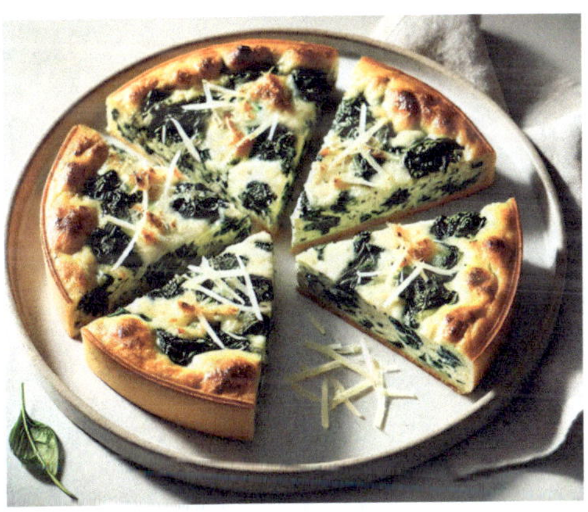

Number of servings: 4

Preparation time: 10 minutes

Cooking time: 25 minutes

Ingredients:

- 6 large eggs
- 1 cup ricotta cheese
- 1 cup fresh spinach, chopped
- 1/2 cup shredded Parmesan cheese
- 1/4 tsp nutmeg (optional)
- 1/4 tsp salt
- 1/4 tsp black pepper

Directions:

1. Preheat the oven to 375°F (190°C) and lightly grease a baking dish.
2. In a large bowl, whisk together the eggs, ricotta cheese, Parmesan, nutmeg, salt, and pepper.
3. Fold in the chopped spinach.
4. Pour the mixture into the prepared baking dish and spread evenly.
5. Bake for 25 minutes or until the top is golden and the center is set.
6. Let cool slightly before slicing and serving.

Nutritional value per serving: Calories: 190, Carbs: 3g, Fiber: 1g, Sugars: 1g, Protein: 13g, Saturated fat: 6g, Unsaturated fat: 4g

Difficulty rating: ★★☆☆☆

Tips for ingredient variations: Add sun-dried tomatoes or cooked sausage for extra flavor. This bake also reheats well for meal prep.

Protein Shake with Peanut Butter and Cocoa

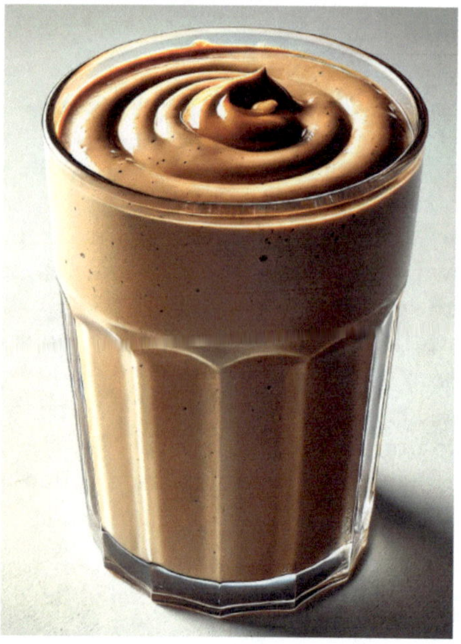

Number of servings: 1

Preparation time: 5 minutes

Cooking time: 0 minutes

Ingredients:

- 1 cup unsweetened almond milk
- 1 scoop chocolate protein powder
- 1 tbsp natural peanut butter
- 1 tsp unsweetened cocoa powder
- 1/4 tsp vanilla extract
- Ice cubes (optional)

Directions:

1. Add all the ingredients to a blender.
2. Blend until smooth, adding ice cubes if a thicker consistency is desired.
3. Pour into a glass and serve immediately.

Nutritional value per serving: Calories: 200, Carbs: 5g, Fiber: 2g, Sugars: 1g, Protein: 20g, Saturated fat: 2g, Unsaturated fat: 6g

Difficulty rating: ★☆☆☆☆

Tips for ingredient variations: Use almond butter instead of peanut butter for a different flavor profile or add a sprinkle of cinnamon for a warm spice note.

Baked Eggs in Avocado Halves

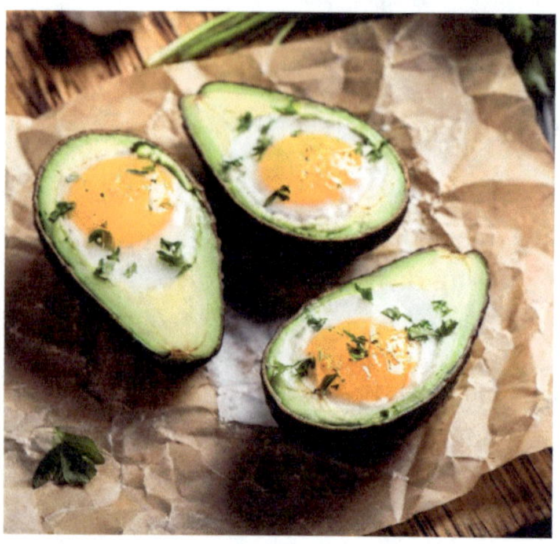

Number of servings: 2

Preparation time: 5 minutes

Cooking time: 15 minutes

Ingredients:

- 1 large avocado, halved and pitted
- 2 large eggs
- Sea salt and black pepper to taste
- 1 tbsp chopped fresh chives or parsley (optional)

Directions:

1. Preheat the oven to 400°F (200°C) and line a baking dish with parchment paper.
2. Scoop out a small portion of avocado flesh to create a larger cavity for the egg.
3. Place the avocado halves in the baking dish and crack one egg into each cavity.
4. Season with salt and pepper.
5. Bake for 12-15 minutes or until the egg whites are set but the yolks remain slightly runny.
6. Garnish with chives or parsley and serve warm.

Nutritional value per serving: Calories: 220, Carbs: 4g, Fiber: 3g, Sugars: 1g, Protein: 8g, Saturated fat: 3g, Unsaturated fat: 14g

Difficulty rating: ★☆☆☆☆

Tips for ingredient variations: Top with a sprinkle of red pepper flakes or shredded cheese for added flavor.

Lunch

Grilled Chicken Salad with Avocado and Olive Oil Dressing

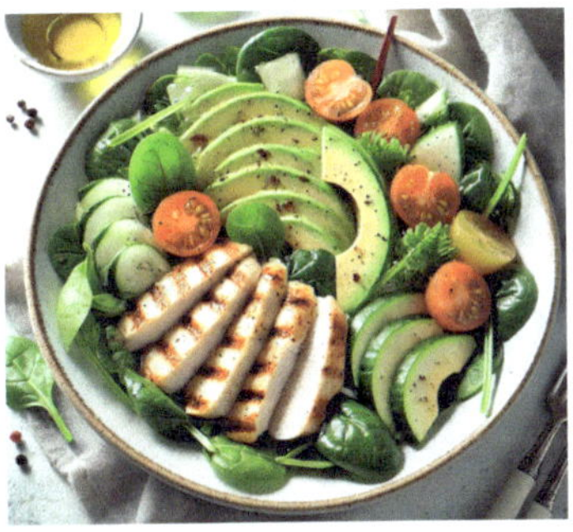

Number of servings: 2

Preparation time: 10 minutes

Cooking time: 15 minutes

Ingredients:

- 2 boneless, skinless chicken breasts
- 1 tbsp olive oil (for grilling the chicken)
- 1 medium avocado, sliced
- 4 cups mixed salad greens (spinach, arugula, romaine)
- 1/2 cup cherry tomatoes, halved
- 1/4 cup cucumber, sliced
- 3 tbsp extra virgin olive oil (for dressing)
- 1 tbsp lemon juice
- Sea salt and black pepper to taste

Directions:

1. Season the chicken breasts with salt and pepper. Heat 1 tbsp olive oil in a grill pan over medium heat and cook the chicken for 6-7 minutes per side, or until fully cooked. Remove from heat and let rest for 5 minutes before slicing.
2. In a large bowl, combine salad greens, cherry tomatoes, cucumber, and avocado.
3. In a small bowl, whisk together 3 tbsp olive oil, lemon juice, salt, and pepper to create the dressing.
4. Add the grilled chicken slices to the salad and drizzle with the dressing. Toss gently to combine.
5. Serve immediately.

Nutritional value per serving: Calories: 320, Carbs: 7g, Fiber: 3g, Sugars: 2g, Protein: 28g, Saturated fat: 4g, Unsaturated fat: 17g

Difficulty rating: ★☆☆☆☆

Tips for ingredient variations: Add sliced almonds or pumpkin seeds for added crunch. Substitute lemon juice with balsamic vinegar for a tangy twist.

Tuna Salad Lettuce Wraps

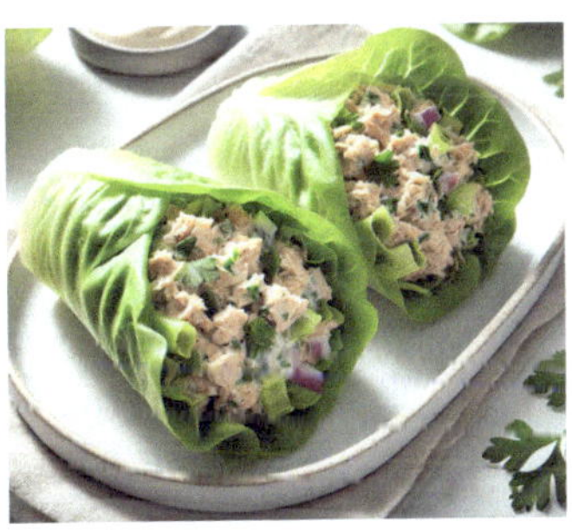

Number of servings: 2

Preparation time: 10 minutes

Cooking time: 0 minutes

Ingredients:

- 1 can (5 oz) tuna in water, drained
- 2 tbsp mayonnaise (or Greek yogurt for a lighter option)
- 1 celery stalk, finely diced
- 1 tbsp red onion, finely chopped
- 1 tbsp fresh parsley, chopped
- 6 large lettuce leaves (e.g., romaine or butter lettuce)
- Sea salt and black pepper to taste

Directions:

1. In a bowl, mix the tuna, mayonnaise, celery, red onion, parsley, salt, and pepper until well combined.
2. Spoon the tuna mixture evenly onto the lettuce leaves.
3. Fold the lettuce around the filling to create wraps and serve immediately.

Nutritional value per serving: Calories: 200, Carbs: 3g, Fiber: 1g, Sugars: 1g, Protein: 22g, Saturated fat: 2g, Unsaturated fat: 6g

Difficulty rating: ★☆☆☆☆

Tips for ingredient variations: Add diced pickles or a squeeze of lemon juice for extra flavor.

Turkey and Cheese Roll-Ups with Spinach

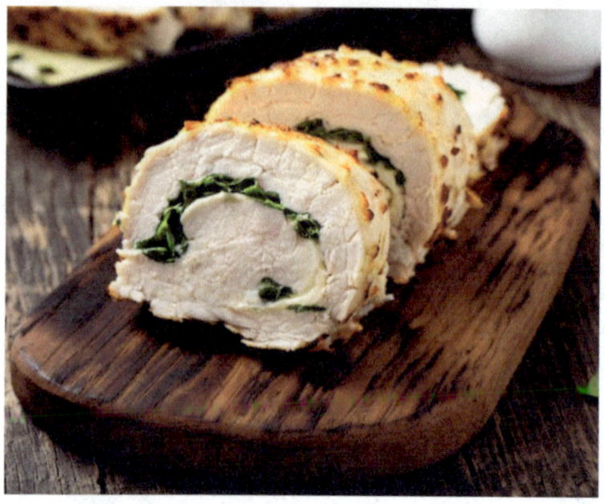

Number of servings: 2

Preparation time: 5 minutes

Cooking time: 0 minutes

Ingredients:

- 6 slices deli turkey (preferably nitrate-free)
- 3 slices Swiss or cheddar cheese, halved
- 1 cup baby spinach leaves
- 1 tbsp mustard or mayonnaise (optional)

Directions:

1. Lay a slice of turkey flat and place half a slice of cheese on top.
2. Add a few spinach leaves on top of the cheese and drizzle with mustard or spread mayonnaise if desired.
3. Roll the turkey tightly around the filling to create a roll-up. Repeat with remaining ingredients.
4. Serve as-is or cut each roll-up into bite-sized pieces.

Nutritional value per serving: Calories: 180, Carbs: 2g, Fiber: 0g, Sugars: 0g, Protein: 20g, Saturated fat: 5g, Unsaturated fat: 3g

Difficulty rating: ★☆☆☆☆

Tips for ingredient variations: Add thinly sliced avocado or cucumber for added texture and flavor.

Zoodles (Zucchini Noodles) with Pesto and Grilled Shrimp

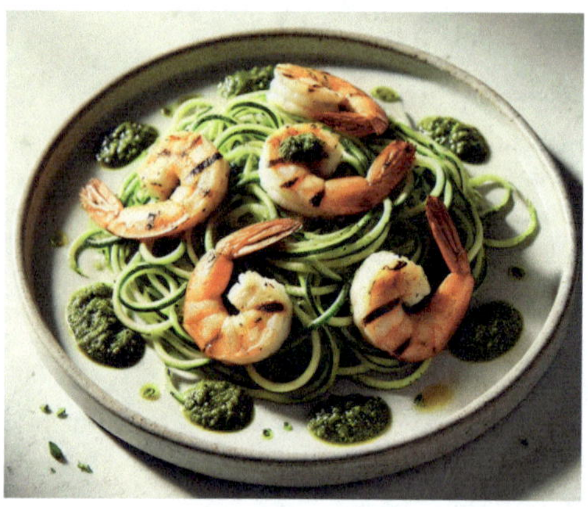

Number of servings: 2

Preparation time: 10 minutes

Cooking time: 10 minutes

Ingredients:

- 2 medium zucchinis, spiralized into noodles
- 1/2 cup basil pesto (store-bought or homemade)
- 12 large shrimp, peeled and deveined
- 1 tbsp olive oil
- Sea salt and black pepper to taste

Directions:

1. Heat olive oil in a skillet over medium heat. Add shrimp, season with salt and pepper, and cook for 2-3 minutes per side until opaque and fully cooked. Remove from heat and set aside.
2. In the same skillet, add the zucchini noodles and sauté for 2-3 minutes until slightly softened.
3. Toss the zoodles with the pesto until evenly coated.
4. Divide the zoodles between two plates and top with the grilled shrimp. Serve immediately.

Nutritional value per serving: Calories: 320, Carbs: 7g, Fiber: 2g, Sugars: 3g, Protein: 25g, Saturated fat: 2g, Unsaturated fat: 8g

Difficulty rating: ★☆☆☆☆

Tips for ingredient variations: Add cherry tomatoes or grated Parmesan for an extra burst of flavor.

Beef and Veggie Stir-Fry (with Coconut Aminos)

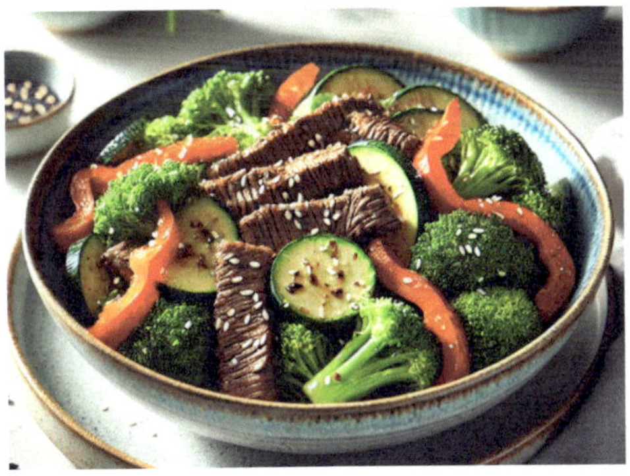

Number of servings: 2
Preparation time: 10 minutes
Cooking time: 15 minutes

Ingredients:

- 8 oz lean beef strips (e.g., sirloin or flank steak)
- 1 cup broccoli florets
- 1 red bell pepper, sliced
- 1 small zucchini, sliced
- 2 tbsp coconut aminos
- 1 tbsp sesame oil or olive oil
- 1 tsp minced garlic
- 1/2 tsp grated ginger
- Sesame seeds for garnish (optional)

Directions:

1. In a big skillet or wok, heat the sesame oil over medium-high heat. Add the beef strips and stir-fry for 3-4 minutes until browned. Remove and set aside.
2. In the same skillet, add garlic and ginger, then stir in broccoli, bell pepper, and zucchini. Cook for 5-7 minutes until vegetables are tender-crisp.
3. Return the beef to the skillet, add coconut aminos, and stir to coat everything evenly. Cook for an additional 2 minutes.
4. Serve hot and garnish with sesame seeds if desired.

Nutritional value per serving: Calories: 280, Carbs: 8g, Fiber: 3g, Sugars: 4g, Protein: 28g, Saturated fat: 4g, Unsaturated fat: 6g

Difficulty rating: ★★☆☆☆

Tips for ingredient variations: Swap beef with chicken or shrimp for variety. Add a splash of lime juice for a tangy finish.

Grilled Salmon with Steamed Broccoli

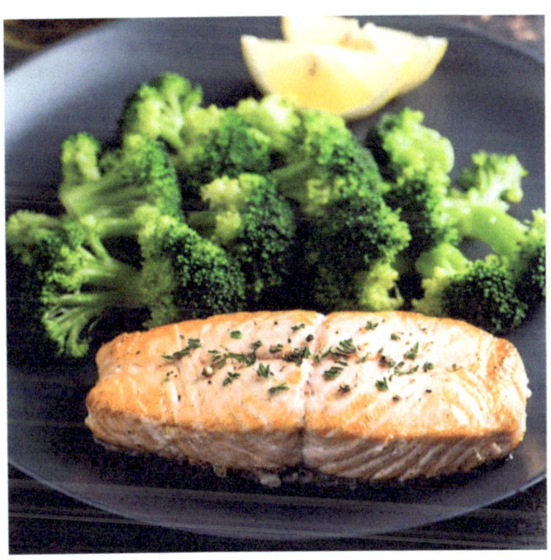

Number of servings: 2
Preparation time: 10 minutes
Cooking time: 15 minutes

Ingredients:

- 2 salmon fillets (6 oz each)
- 2 cups fresh broccoli florets
- 1 tbsp olive oil
- 1 clove garlic, minced
- 1/2 lemon, sliced
- Sea salt and black pepper to taste

Directions:

1. Preheat the grill or grill pan over medium heat.
2. Brush the salmon fillets with olive oil and season with garlic, salt, and pepper.
3. Make sure the salmon flakes easily with a fork after grilling it for 4–5 minutes on each side.
4. Meanwhile, steam the broccoli florets in a pot with a steamer basket over boiling water for 5-7 minutes until tender.
5. Serve the grilled salmon with steamed broccoli, garnished with lemon slices.

Nutritional value per serving: Calories: 310, Carbs: 6g, Fiber: 3g, Sugars: 2g, Protein: 34g, Saturated fat: 2g, Unsaturated fat: 9g

Difficulty rating: ★☆☆☆☆

Tips for ingredient variations: Add a sprinkle of red pepper flakes to the salmon for a spicy kick, or toss the broccoli with a drizzle of soy sauce and sesame seeds for extra flavor.

Greek Salad with Feta and Grilled Chicken

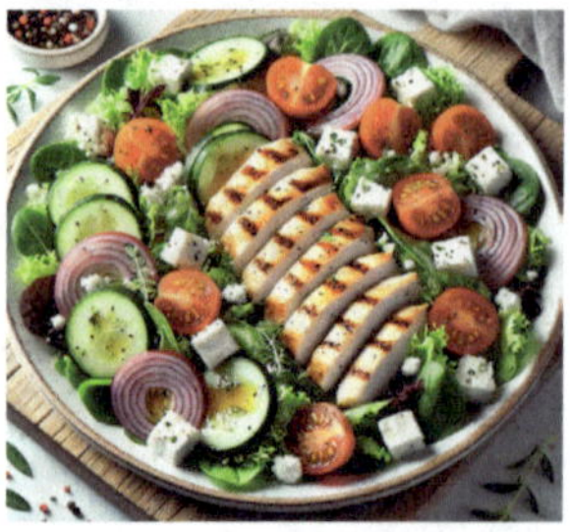

Number of servings: 2

Preparation time: 15 minutes

Cooking time: 10 minutes

Ingredients:

- 2 cups mixed greens (spinach, arugula, and romaine)
- 1 cup cherry tomatoes, halved
- 1/2 cucumber, sliced
- 1/4 cup red onion, thinly sliced
- 1/4 cup crumbled feta cheese
- 2 grilled chicken breasts (6 oz each), sliced
- 2 tbsp olive oil
- 1 tbsp red wine vinegar
- 1/2 tsp dried oregano
- Sea salt and black pepper to taste

Directions:

1. Preheat the grill or grill pan to medium-high heat. Season the chicken breasts with salt, pepper, and a sprinkle of oregano. Grill for 4-5 minutes on each side or until fully cooked. Let rest, then slice.
2. Add the mixed greens, cucumber, red onion, cherry tomatoes, and feta cheese to a large salad dish.
3. Mix the olive oil, red wine vinegar, oregano, salt, and pepper in a small bowl.
4. Drizzle the dressing over the salad and toss gently to coat.
5. Top the salad with grilled chicken slices and serve.

Nutritional value per serving: Calories: 340, Carbs: 10g, Fiber: 3g, Sugars: 4g, Protein: 38g, Saturated fat: 4g, Unsaturated fat: 12g

Difficulty rating: ★☆☆☆☆

Tips for ingredient variations: Swap feta with goat cheese or add Kalamata olives for a more traditional Greek flavor.

Low-Carb Turkey Chili

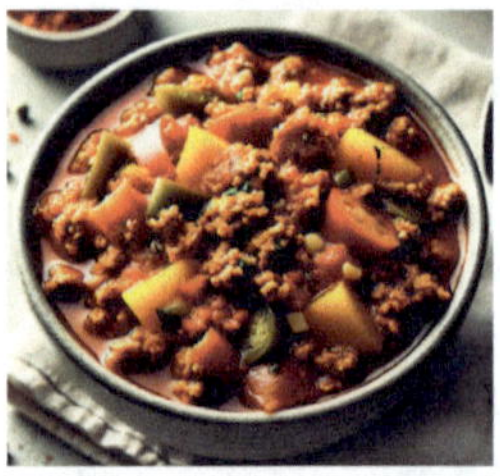

Number of servings: 4

Preparation time: 10 minutes

Cooking time: 25 minutes

Ingredients:

- 1 lb ground turkey
- 1 cup diced tomatoes (canned or fresh)
- 1 cup bell peppers, diced
- 1/2 cup onion, diced
- 1 cup chicken broth
- 2 tbsp tomato paste
- 1 tsp chili powder
- 1 tsp cumin
- 1/2 tsp smoked paprika
- 1 tbsp olive oil
- Sea salt and black pepper to taste

Directions:

1. Heat olive oil in a large pot over medium heat. Add the onion and bell peppers, cooking for 3-4 minutes until softened.
2. Add the ground turkey and cook until browned, breaking it up with a spoon.
3. Stir in diced tomatoes, tomato paste, chicken broth, chili powder, cumin, paprika, salt, and pepper.
4. Bring the chili to a boil, then reduce the heat to low and simmer for 20 minutes, stirring occasionally.
5. Serve hot, garnished with fresh cilantro or a dollop of Greek yogurt, if desired.

Nutritional value per serving: Calories: 250, Carbs: 8g, Fiber: 3g, Sugars: 3g, Protein: 28g, Saturated fat: 2g, Unsaturated fat: 5g

Difficulty rating: ★☆☆☆☆

Tips for ingredient variations: Add diced zucchini or spinach for extra vegetables, or use ground chicken as a substitute for turkey.

BLT Lettuce Wraps

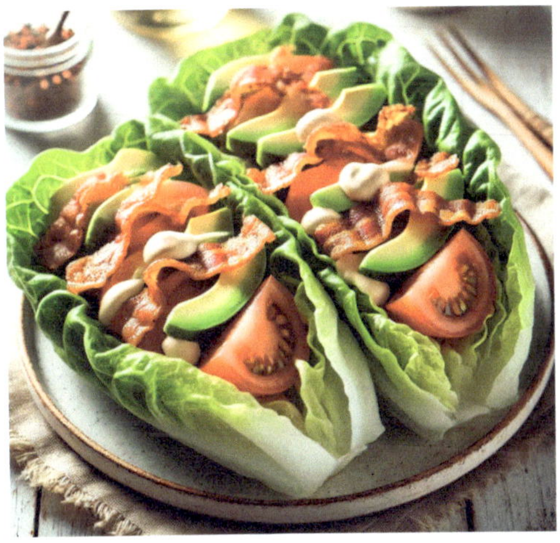

Number of servings: 2

Preparation time: 10 minutes

Cooking time: 10 minutes

Ingredients:

- 4 large leaves of iceberg or romaine lettuce
- 4 slices cooked bacon
- 1 small tomato, sliced
- 1/2 avocado, sliced
- 1/4 cup mayonnaise
- Sea salt and black pepper to taste

Directions:

1. Lay the lettuce leaves flat and spread a thin layer of mayonnaise on each.
2. Add slices of tomato, avocado, and two strips of bacon to each leaf.
3. Season with salt and pepper, then fold the lettuce leaves into wraps.
4. Secure with toothpicks if needed and serve immediately.

Nutritional value per serving: Calories: 220, Carbs: 5g, Fiber: 3g, Sugars: 2g, Protein: 10g, Saturated fat: 4g, Unsaturated fat: 9g

Difficulty rating: ★☆☆☆☆

Tips for ingredient variations: Add grilled chicken or turkey slices for extra protein, or drizzle with hot sauce for added spice.

Egg Salad with Low-Carb Crackers

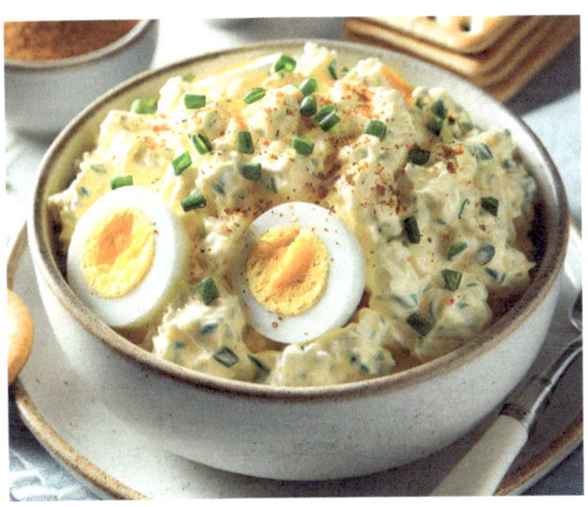

Number of servings: 2

Preparation time: 10 minutes

Cooking time: 10 minutes

Ingredients:

- 4 hard-boiled eggs, chopped
- 2 tbsp mayonnaise
- 1 tsp Dijon mustard
- 1 tbsp chopped chives
- 1/4 tsp paprika
- Sea salt and black pepper to taste
- 8-10 low-carb crackers

Directions:

1. In a bowl, combine the chopped eggs, mayonnaise, Dijon mustard, chives, paprika, salt, and pepper. Mix until well combined.
2. Serve the egg salad with low-carb crackers on the side or use the crackers to scoop the salad.

Nutritional value per serving: Calories: 190, Carbs: 4g, Fiber: 1g, Sugars: 1g, Protein: 12g, Saturated fat: 3g, Unsaturated fat: 6g

Difficulty rating: ★☆☆☆☆

Tips for ingredient variations: Add diced celery or pickles for added crunch, or use Greek yogurt in place of mayonnaise for a lighter option.

Pulled Pork Salad Bowl

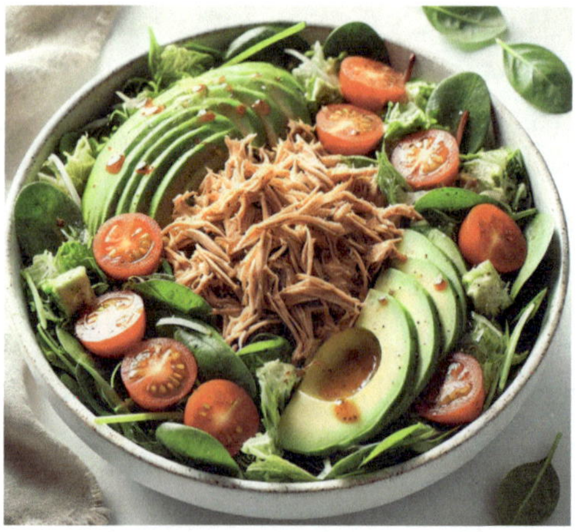

Number of servings: 2

Preparation time: 10 minutes

Cooking time: 0 minutes

Ingredients:

- 2 cups shredded pulled pork (cooked, no added sugar or barbecue sauce)
- 4 cups mixed salad greens
- 1/2 cup cherry tomatoes, halved
- 1/2 avocado, sliced
- 2 tbsp olive oil
- 1 tbsp apple cider vinegar
- 1 tsp Dijon mustard
- Sea salt and black pepper to taste

Directions:

1. In a large bowl, combine the salad greens, cherry tomatoes, and avocado slices.
2. Add the pulled pork on top of the greens.
3. In a small bowl, whisk together the olive oil, apple cider vinegar, Dijon mustard, salt, and pepper.
4. Drizzle the dressing over the salad and toss gently to combine.
5. Serve immediately.

Nutritional value per serving: Calories: 320, Carbs: 6g, Fiber: 3g, Sugars: 2g, Protein: 22g, Saturated fat: 3g, Unsaturated fat: 14g

Difficulty rating: ★☆☆☆☆

Tips for ingredient variations: Add shredded cheese or chopped nuts for extra flavor and crunch.

Steak Salad with Blue Cheese Crumbles

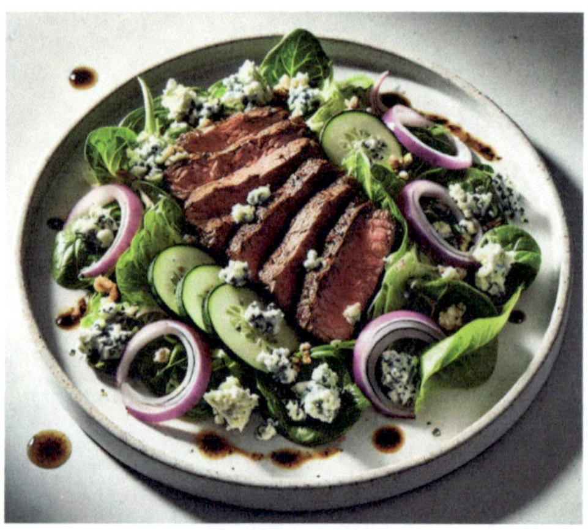

Number of servings: 2

Preparation time: 10 minutes

Cooking time: 10 minutes

Ingredients:

- 200g flank steak, cooked to preference and sliced
- 4 cups mixed greens
- 1/4 cup blue cheese crumbles
- 1/2 cup cucumber, sliced
- 1/4 cup red onion, thinly sliced
- 2 tbsp olive oil
- 1 tbsp balsamic vinegar
- Sea salt and black pepper to taste

Directions:

1. Arrange the mixed greens, cucumber, and red onion on two plates.
2. Add the sliced steak on top of the salad.
3. Sprinkle with blue cheese crumbles.
4. In a small bowl, whisk together olive oil, balsamic vinegar, salt, and pepper.
5. Drizzle the dressing over the salad and serve.

Nutritional value per serving: Calories: 310, Carbs: 5g, Fiber: 2g, Sugars: 2g, Protein: 27g, Saturated fat: 6g, Unsaturated fat: 12g

Difficulty rating: ★☆☆☆☆

Tips for ingredient variations: Replace blue cheese with feta or goat cheese for a milder flavor.

Cauliflower Fried Rice with Chicken

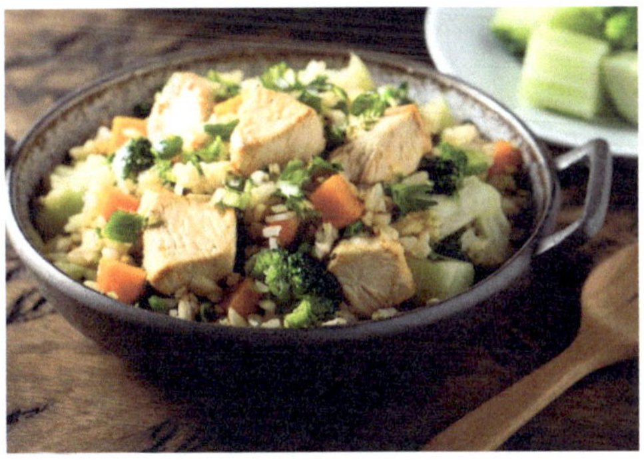

Number of servings: 2

Preparation time: 10 minutes

Cooking time: 10 minutes

Ingredients:

- 2 cups cauliflower rice
- 1 chicken breast, diced and cooked
- 1/2 cup mixed vegetables (carrots, peas, optional)
- 2 large eggs, beaten
- 2 tbsp soy sauce or tamari
- 1 tbsp sesame oil
- 1 clove garlic, minced
- 1 tsp grated ginger
- 2 green onions, sliced

Directions:

1. Heat sesame oil in a large skillet over medium heat.
2. Add garlic and ginger and sauté for 1 minute.
3. Add the cauliflower rice and mixed vegetables, cooking until softened (about 5 minutes).
4. Push the mixture to one side of the skillet and scramble the beaten eggs on the other side until cooked.
5. Stir in the cooked chicken and soy sauce. Mix everything thoroughly.
6. Top with sliced green onions and serve hot.

Nutritional value per serving: Calories: 250, Carbs: 8g, Fiber: 3g, Sugars: 3g, Protein: 28g, Saturated fat: 2g, Unsaturated fat: 7g

Difficulty rating: ★★☆☆☆

Tips for ingredient variations: Add sesame seeds or sriracha for extra flavor and heat.

Baked Cod with Asparagus

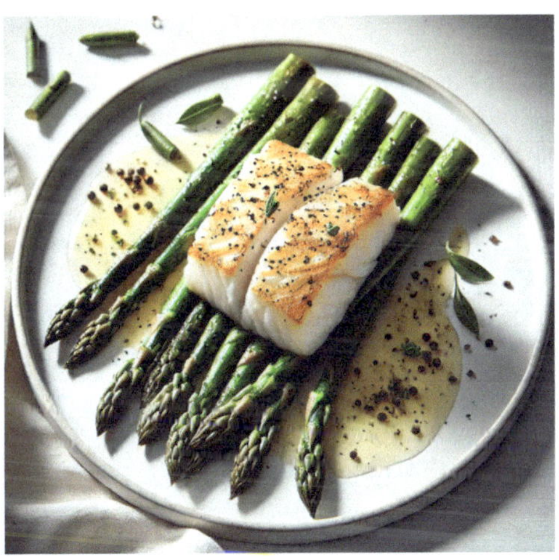

Number of servings: 2

Preparation time: 10 minutes

Cooking time: 20 minutes

Ingredients:

- 2 cod fillets (150g each)
- 200g asparagus, trimmed
- 2 tbsp olive oil
- 1 tbsp lemon juice
- 1 tsp garlic powder
- 1/2 tsp paprika
- Sea salt and black pepper to taste

Directions:

1. Preheat the oven to 375°F (190°C).
2. Arrange cod fillets and asparagus on a lined baking sheet.
3. Drizzle olive oil and lemon juice over the cod and asparagus.
4. Season the fish with salt, pepper, paprika, and garlic powder.
5. The asparagus should be soft and the fish should flake easily with a fork after 18 to 20 minutes of baking.
6. Serve immediately.

Nutritional value per serving: Calories: 200, Carbs: 4g, Fiber: 2g, Sugars: 2g, Protein: 26g, Saturated fat: 2g, Unsaturated fat: 6g

Difficulty rating: ★☆☆☆☆

Tips for ingredient variations: Add fresh dill or parsley for an herbal garnish.

Turkey Meatballs with Tomato Sauce

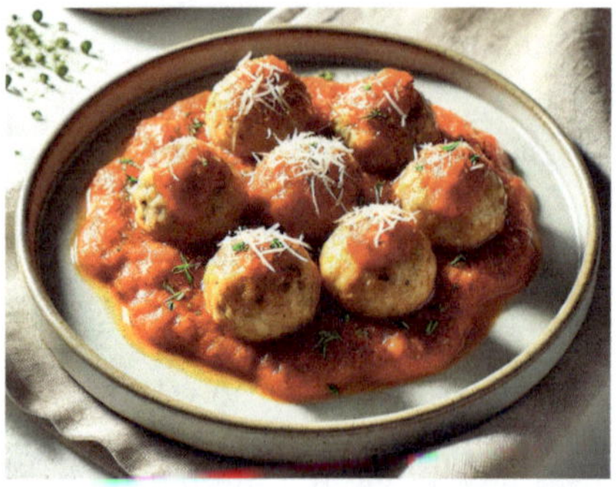

Number of servings: 4 (4 meatballs per serving)
Preparation time: 10 minutes
Cooking time: 25 minutes

Ingredients:

- 500g ground turkey
- 1/4 cup almond flour
- 1 large egg
- 2 garlic cloves, minced
- 1 tsp Italian seasoning
- 1/4 cup grated Parmesan cheese
- 1 can (400g) crushed tomatoes (unsweetened)
- 1 tbsp olive oil
- Sea salt and black pepper to taste

Directions:

1. Preheat oven to 375°F (190°C) and line a baking sheet with parchment paper.
2. In a large bowl, mix ground turkey, almond flour, egg, garlic, Italian seasoning, Parmesan, salt, and pepper until well combined.
3. Shape the mixture into small meatballs and place them on the prepared baking sheet.
4. Bake for 20 minutes or until cooked through.
5. While the meatballs bake, heat olive oil in a saucepan over medium heat. Add crushed tomatoes, season with salt and pepper, and simmer for 5-7 minutes.
6. Toss the baked meatballs in the tomato sauce before serving.

Nutritional value per serving: Calories: 240, Carbs: 6g, Fiber: 2g, Sugars: 2g, Protein: 30g, Saturated fat: 3g, Unsaturated fat: 5g

Difficulty rating: ★★☆☆☆

Tips for ingredient variations: Serve over zucchini noodles or cauliflower rice for a complete meal.

Caprese Salad with Grilled Chicken

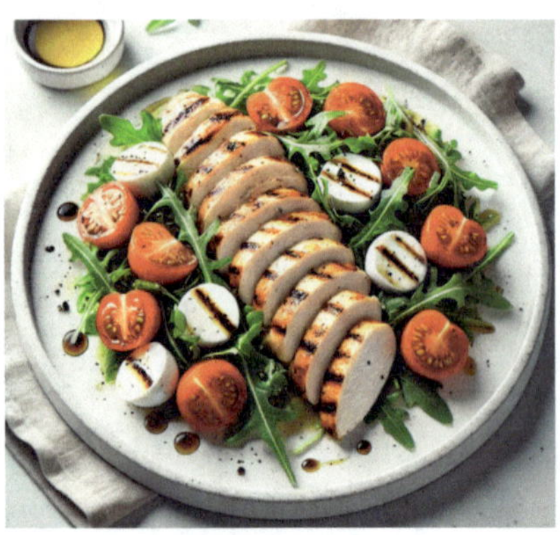

Number of servings: 2
Preparation time: 10 minutes
Cooking time: 15 minutes

Ingredients:

- 2 boneless, skinless chicken breasts
- 2 cups fresh arugula or spinach
- 1 cup cherry tomatoes, halved
- 4 oz fresh mozzarella, sliced
- 1 tbsp extra virgin olive oil
- 1 tbsp balsamic vinegar
- 1 tsp dried oregano
- Sea salt and black pepper to taste

Directions:

1. Preheat a grill or grill pan over medium heat. Season chicken breasts with salt, pepper, and oregano.
2. Grill chicken for 6-8 minutes per side, or until fully cooked and juices run clear. Remove from heat and let rest for 5 minutes.
3. Arrange arugula, cherry tomatoes, and mozzarella slices on a serving plate.
4. Slice the grilled chicken and place it on top of the salad.
5. Drizzle with olive oil and balsamic vinegar, then season with additional salt and pepper to taste. Serve immediately.

Nutritional value per serving: Calories: 320, Carbs: 6g, Fiber: 2g, Sugars: 3g, Protein: 38g, Saturated fat: 6g, Unsaturated fat: 9g

Difficulty rating: ★☆☆☆☆

Tips for ingredient variations: Substitute arugula with mixed greens or add a handful of fresh basil for extra flavor.

Low-Carb Chicken Wraps (Using Lettuce or Collard Greens)

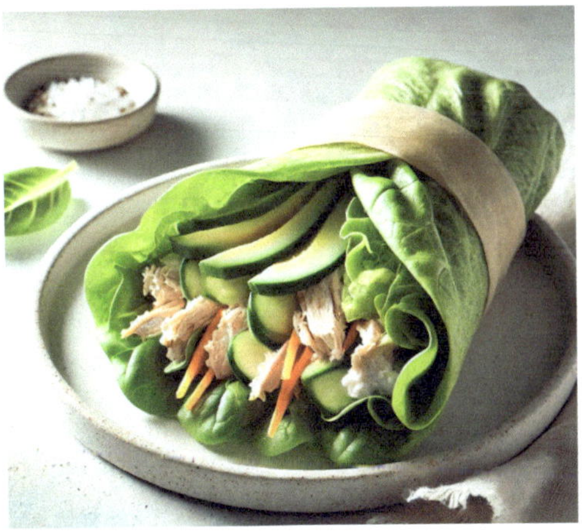

Number of servings: 2

Preparation time: 10 minutes

Cooking time: 10 minutes

Ingredients:

- 2 large lettuce leaves or collard green leaves
- 1 cup cooked, shredded chicken breast
- 1/2 avocado, sliced
- 1/2 cup cucumber, julienned
- 1/4 cup shredded carrots
- 2 tbsp Greek yogurt or hummus
- 1 tsp lemon juice
- Sea salt and black pepper to taste

Directions:

1. Lay the lettuce or collard green leaves flat on a clean surface.
2. Spread a thin layer of Greek yogurt or hummus over each leaf.
3. Top with shredded chicken, avocado slices, cucumber, and carrots.
4. Sprinkle with lemon juice, salt, and pepper.
5. Roll tightly and secure with a toothpick if needed. Serve immediately.

Nutritional value per serving: Calories: 220, Carbs: 5g, Fiber: 3g, Sugars: 1g, Protein: 25g, Saturated fat: 3g, Unsaturated fat: 8g

Difficulty rating: ★☆☆☆☆

Tips for ingredient variations: Add sliced bell peppers or swap Greek yogurt with mashed avocado for a creamier wrap.

Lemon Garlic Shrimp over Cauliflower Mash

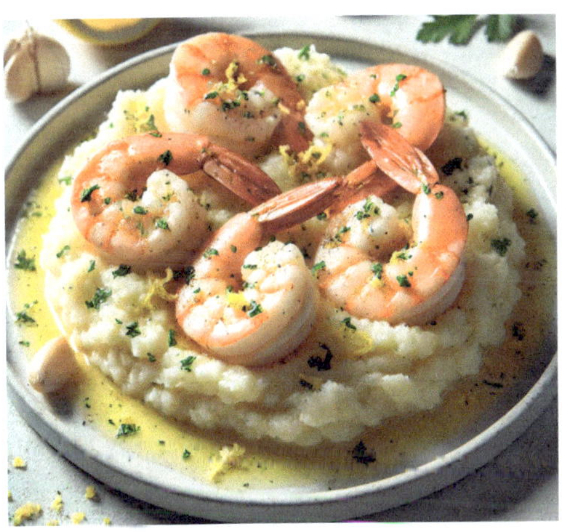

Number of servings: 2

Preparation time: 10 minutes

Cooking time: 20 minutes

Ingredients:

- 12 large shrimp, peeled and deveined
- 2 cups cauliflower florets
- 1 tbsp butter
- 2 tbsp olive oil
- 1 garlic clove, minced
- 1 tsp lemon zest
- 1 tbsp fresh parsley, chopped
- Sea salt and black pepper to taste

Directions:

1. Steam the cauliflower florets until tender, about 10 minutes. Mash with butter, salt, and pepper until smooth. Set aside.
2. Heat olive oil in a skillet over medium heat. Add garlic and sauté for 1 minute until fragrant.
3. Cook the shrimp in the skillet for two to three minutes on each side, or until they are opaque and pink.
4. Stir in lemon zest and parsley.
5. Serve the shrimp over the cauliflower mash, drizzling the garlic-infused oil from the skillet on top.

Nutritional value per serving: Calories: 290, Carbs: 7g, Fiber: 3g, Sugars: 2g, Protein: 25g, Saturated fat: 4g, Unsaturated fat: 12g

Difficulty rating: ★★☆☆☆

Tips for ingredient variations: Add a splash of chicken stock to the cauliflower mash for extra flavor.

Grilled Sausage with Roasted Peppers

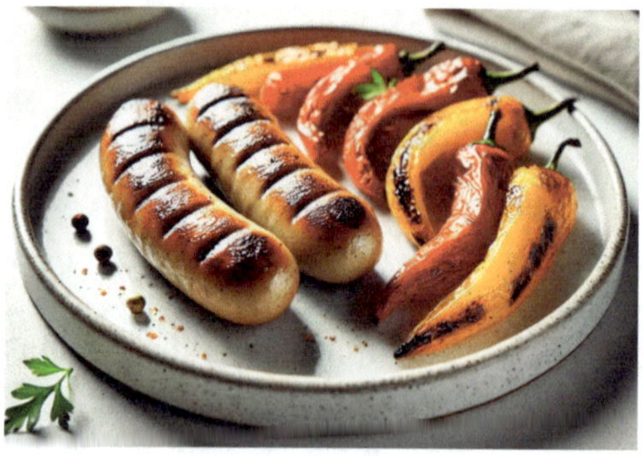

Number of servings: 2

Preparation time: 10 minutes

Cooking time: 20 minutes

Ingredients:

- 4 chicken or turkey sausages
- 1 red bell pepper, sliced
- 1 yellow bell pepper, sliced
- 1 tbsp olive oil
- 1 tsp smoked paprika
- Sea salt and black pepper to taste

Directions:

1. Preheat a grill or grill pan over medium heat. Grill sausages for 10-12 minutes, turning occasionally, until fully cooked.
2. In the meantime, toss bell pepper slices with olive oil, smoked paprika, salt, and pepper.
3. Roast the peppers in a preheated oven at 375°F (190°C) for 15 minutes or until tender and slightly charred.
4. Serve grilled sausages alongside the roasted peppers.

Nutritional value per serving: Calories: 310, Carbs: 8g, Fiber: 2g, Sugars: 4g, Protein: 24g, Saturated fat: 3g, Unsaturated fat: 8g

Difficulty rating: ★☆☆☆☆

Tips for ingredient variations: Add zucchini or mushrooms to the roasted peppers for additional vegetables.

Sesame Ginger Chicken Stir-Fry

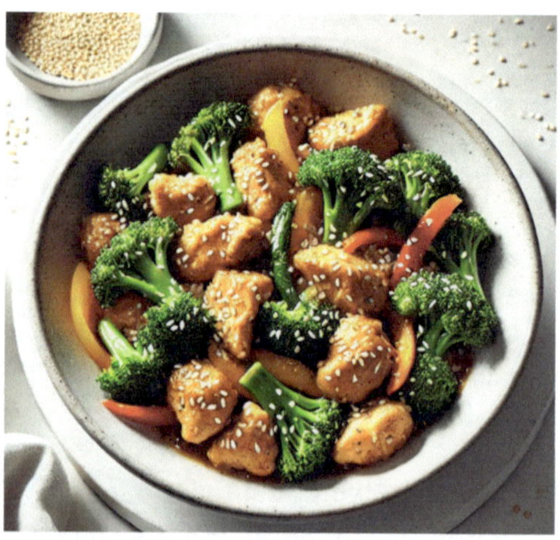

Number of servings: 2

Preparation time: 10 minutes

Cooking time: 15 minutes

Ingredients:

- 2 boneless, skinless chicken breasts, diced
- 1 cup broccoli florets
- 1/2 cup bell peppers, sliced
- 1/4 cup soy sauce or coconut aminos
- 1 tbsp sesame oil
- 1 tsp grated ginger
- 1 garlic clove, minced
- 1 tsp sesame seeds
- Sea salt and black pepper to taste

Directions:

1. In a big skillet or wok, heat the sesame oil over medium-high heat.
2. Add diced chicken and cook for 5-7 minutes, stirring occasionally, until golden brown and cooked through. Remove from the skillet and set aside.
3. In the same skillet, add broccoli and bell peppers. Cook for 5 minutes until tender-crisp.
4. Return the chicken to the skillet and stir in soy sauce, ginger, and garlic. Cook for 2-3 minutes until well combined and heated through.
5. Sprinkle with sesame seeds and serve immediately.

Nutritional value per serving: Calories: 280, Carbs: 8g, Fiber: 2g, Sugars: 3g, Protein: 35g, Saturated fat: 2g, Unsaturated fat: 7g

Difficulty rating: ★★☆☆☆

Tips for ingredient variations: Add mushrooms or zucchini to the stir-fry for more vegetables. Use chili flakes for a spicy kick.

Spinach and Tuna Salad with Lemon Dressing

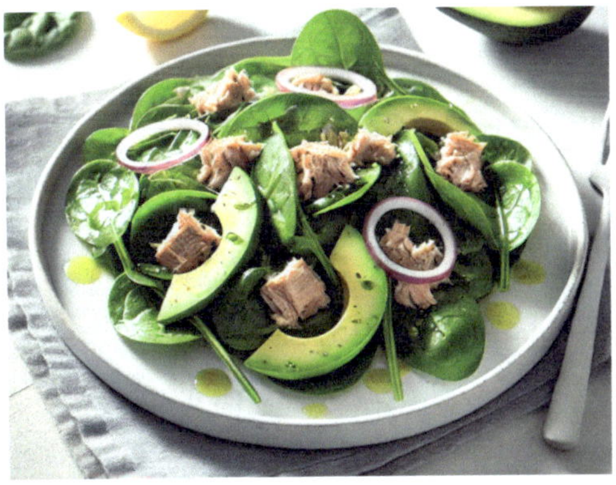

Number of servings: 2

Preparation time: 10 minutes

Cooking time: 0 minutes

Ingredients:

- 2 cups fresh spinach
- 1 can (5 oz) tuna in water, drained
- 1/2 avocado, sliced
- 1/4 cup red onion, thinly sliced
- 2 tbsp olive oil
- 1 tbsp lemon juice
- 1 tsp Dijon mustard
- Sea salt and black pepper to taste

Directions:

1. In a large salad bowl, combine spinach, tuna, avocado slices, and red onion.
2. Add the lemon juice, Dijon mustard, olive oil, salt, and pepper to a small bowl and mix well.
3. Drizzle the dressing over the salad and toss gently to combine.
4. Serve immediately.

Nutritional value per serving: Calories: 230, Carbs: 4g, Fiber: 2g, Sugars: 1g, Protein: 20g, Saturated fat: 3g, Unsaturated fat: 15g

Difficulty rating: ★☆☆☆☆

Tips for ingredient variations: Add boiled eggs or cucumber slices for extra texture and protein.

Zucchini Lasagna (Layered with Ricotta and Ground Turkey)

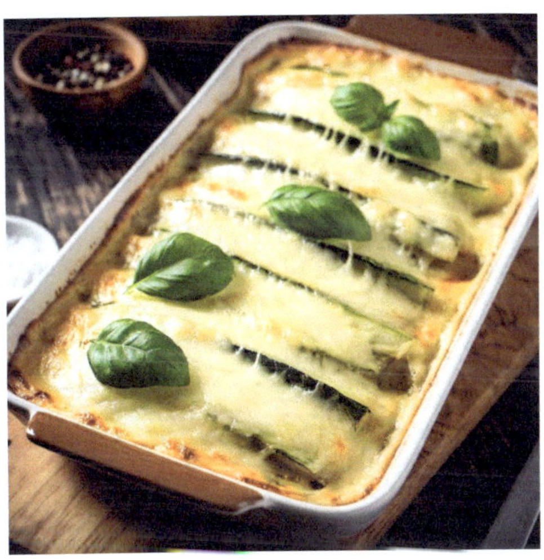

Number of servings: 4

Preparation time: 20 minutes

Cooking time: 40 minutes

Ingredients:

- 3 medium zucchinis, sliced lengthwise into thin strips
- 1 lb ground turkey
- 1 cup ricotta cheese
- 1 cup shredded mozzarella cheese
- 1 cup marinara sauce (sugar-free)
- 1 tbsp olive oil
- 2 garlic cloves, minced
- 1 tsp dried oregano
- 1 tsp dried basil
- Sea salt and black pepper to taste

Directions:

1. Preheat oven to 375°F (190°C).
2. Heat olive oil in a skillet over medium heat. Add garlic and sauté for 1 minute. Add ground turkey and cook until browned. Season with oregano, basil, salt, and pepper.
3. Spread a thin layer of marinara sauce in a baking dish. Layer zucchini strips, turkey mixture, ricotta, and marinara sauce. Repeat until ingredients are used, ending with a layer of zucchini topped with mozzarella.
4. Bake for 35-40 minutes, or until the cheese is melted and bubbly.
5. Let rest for 5 minutes before serving.

Nutritional value per serving: Calories: 310, Carbs: 6g, Fiber: 2g, Sugars: 2g, Protein: 28g, Saturated fat: 7g, Unsaturated fat: 9g

Difficulty rating: ★★☆☆☆

Tips for ingredient variations: Use ground chicken or beef instead of turkey. Add spinach or mushrooms for extra vegetables.

Grilled Steak with Garlic Butter Mushrooms

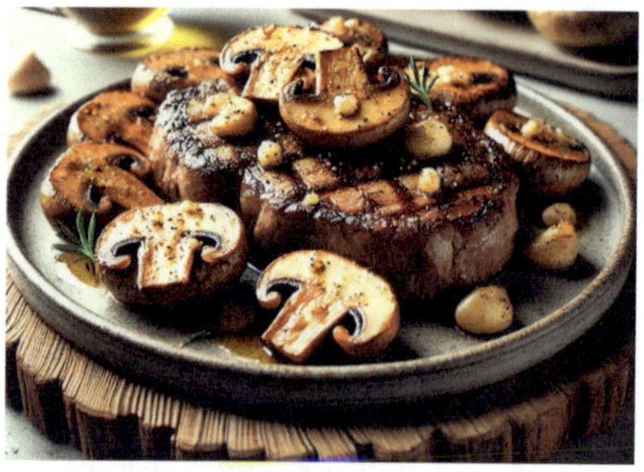

Number of servings: 2
Preparation time: 10 minutes
Cooking time: 15 minutes

Ingredients:

- 2 (6 oz) sirloin steaks
- 1 cup mushrooms, sliced
- 2 tbsp butter
- 1 garlic clove, minced
- 1 tbsp olive oil
- Sea salt and black pepper to taste

Directions:

1. Heat a grill or skillet over medium-high heat. Season steaks with salt and pepper.
2. Grill steaks for 3-4 minutes per side for medium-rare, or until desired doneness. Remove and let rest.
3. In a skillet, heat olive oil and butter. Add garlic and sauté for 1 minute. Add mushrooms and cook until tender.
4. Serve steaks topped with garlic butter mushrooms.

Nutritional value per serving: Calories: 340, Carbs: 3g, Fiber: 1g, Sugars: 1g, Protein: 35g, Saturated fat: 10g, Unsaturated fat: 8g

Difficulty rating: ★☆☆☆☆

Tips for ingredient variations: Add a sprinkle of fresh parsley or serve with a side of roasted asparagus.

Chicken Caesar Salad (Without Croutons)

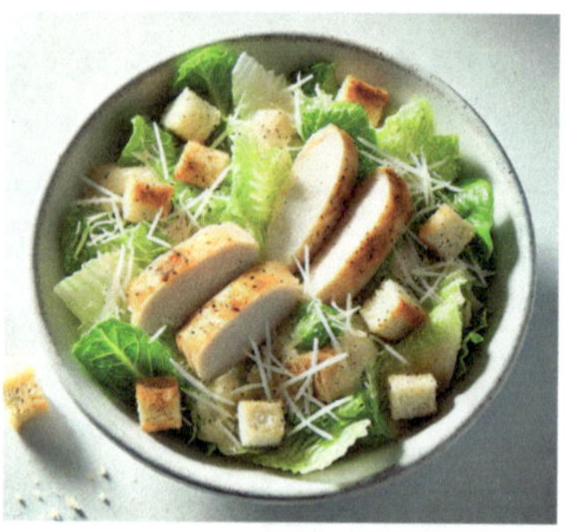

Number of servings: 2
Preparation time: 10 minutes
Cooking time: 10 minutes

Ingredients:

- 2 cups romaine lettuce, chopped
- 1 grilled chicken breast, sliced
- 1/4 cup grated Parmesan cheese
- 2 tbsp Caesar dressing (low-carb)
- 1 tbsp olive oil
- Sea salt and black pepper to taste

Directions:

1. In a large bowl, combine romaine lettuce, sliced chicken, and Parmesan cheese.
2. Drizzle with Caesar dressing and toss gently to coat.
3. Serve immediately.

Nutritional value per serving: Calories: 290, Carbs: 4g, Fiber: 1g, Sugars: 1g, Protein: 30g, Saturated fat: 5g, Unsaturated fat: 10g

Difficulty rating: ★☆☆☆☆

Tips for ingredient variations: Add a soft-boiled egg or avocado slices for extra richness.

Avocado Egg Salad Bowl

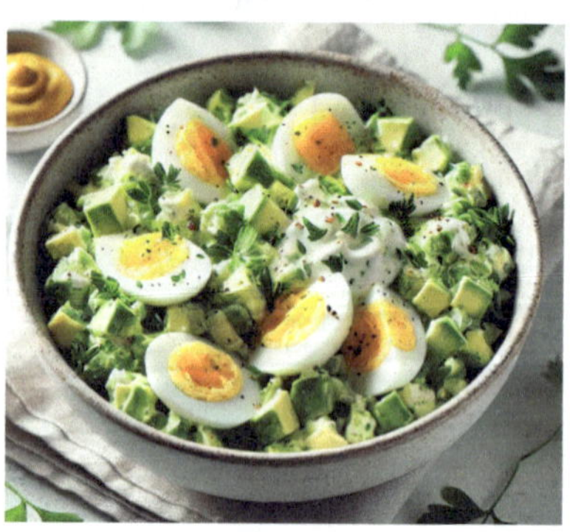

Number of servings: 2
Preparation time: 10 minutes
Cooking time: 10 minutes

Ingredients:

- 4 large eggs, hard-boiled and chopped
- 1 avocado, diced
- 1 tbsp Greek yogurt (optional)
- 1 tsp Dijon mustard
- 1 tbsp fresh parsley, chopped
- Sea salt and black pepper to taste

Directions:

1. In a bowl, combine chopped eggs, avocado, and Greek yogurt.
2. Add Dijon mustard, parsley, salt, and pepper. Mix gently until well combined.
3. Serve in bowls and enjoy.

Nutritional value per serving: Calories: 220, Carbs: 5g, Fiber: 3g, Sugars: 1g, Protein: 12g, Saturated fat: 3g, Unsaturated fat: 15g

Difficulty rating: ★☆☆☆☆

Tips for ingredient variations: Serve over a bed of mixed greens or with cucumber slices for added crunch.

Dinner

Baked Chicken Thighs with Brussels Sprouts

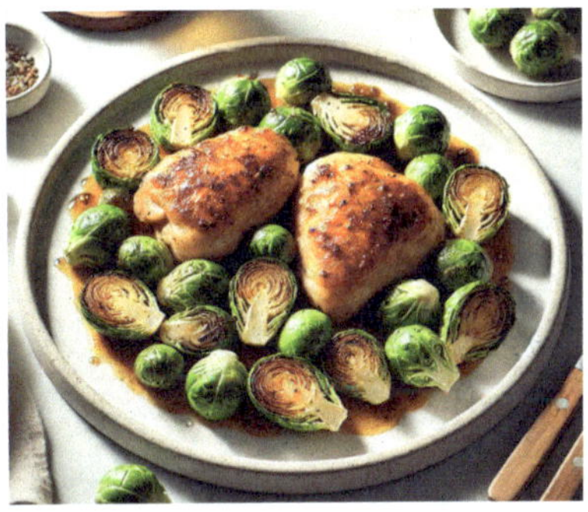

Number of servings: 4

Preparation time: 10 minutes

Cooking time: 30 minutes

Ingredients:

- 4 chicken thighs (bone-in, skin-on)
- 2 cups Brussels sprouts, halved
- 2 tbsp olive oil
- 2 garlic cloves, minced
- 1 tsp paprika
- 1 tsp dried thyme
- Sea salt and black pepper to taste

Directions:

1. Preheat the oven to 400°F (200°C).
2. In a bowl, toss the Brussels sprouts with 1 tablespoon of olive oil, half the minced garlic, salt, and pepper. Spread them on a baking sheet.
3. Pat the chicken thighs dry and rub with the remaining olive oil, paprika, thyme, and garlic. Season with salt and pepper.
4. Place the chicken thighs on the baking sheet with the Brussels sprouts.
5. Bake for 30 minutes or until the chicken skin is crispy and the internal temperature reaches 165°F (74°C).
6. Serve hot and enjoy.

Nutritional value per serving: Calories: 320, Carbs: 7g, Fiber: 3g, Sugars: 2g, Protein: 24g, Saturated fat: 3g, Unsaturated fat: 11g

Difficulty rating: ★☆☆☆☆

Tips for ingredient variations: Add a sprinkle of Parmesan to the Brussels sprouts for extra flavor.

Garlic Butter Salmon with Green Beans

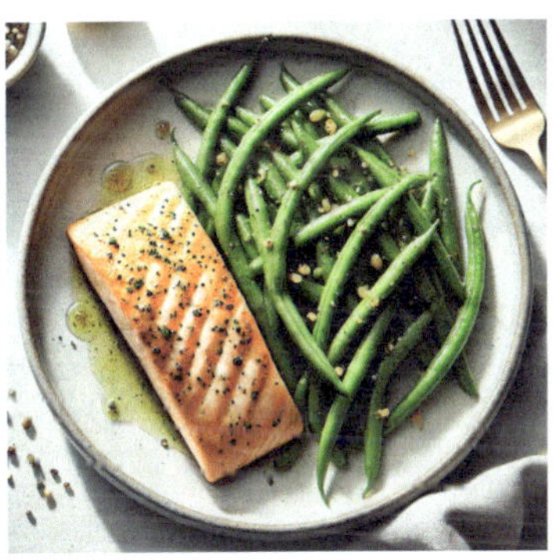

Number of servings: 2

Preparation time: 10 minutes

Cooking time: 15 minutes

Ingredients:

- 2 salmon fillets (about 6 oz each)
- 2 cups green beans, trimmed
- 2 tbsp butter
- 3 garlic cloves, minced
- 1 tbsp lemon juice
- Sea salt and black pepper to taste

Directions:

1. Preheat a skillet over medium heat and add 1 tablespoon of butter.
2. After adding salt and pepper to the salmon fillets, put them on the skillet skin-side down. Cook for 4-5 minutes, then flip and cook for another 2-3 minutes. Remove and set aside.
3. In the same skillet, add the remaining butter and minced garlic. Sauté for 30 seconds, then add the green beans.
4. Cook the green beans for 4-5 minutes, stirring occasionally. Drizzle with lemon juice.
5. Serve the salmon alongside the garlic butter green beans.

Nutritional value per serving: Calories: 380, Carbs: 5g, Fiber: 2g, Sugars: 1g, Protein: 32g, Saturated fat: 6g, Unsaturated fat: 11g

Difficulty rating: ★☆☆☆☆

Tips for ingredient variations: Add red pepper flakes for a bit of heat.

Low-Carb Beef Tacos (with Lettuce Wraps)

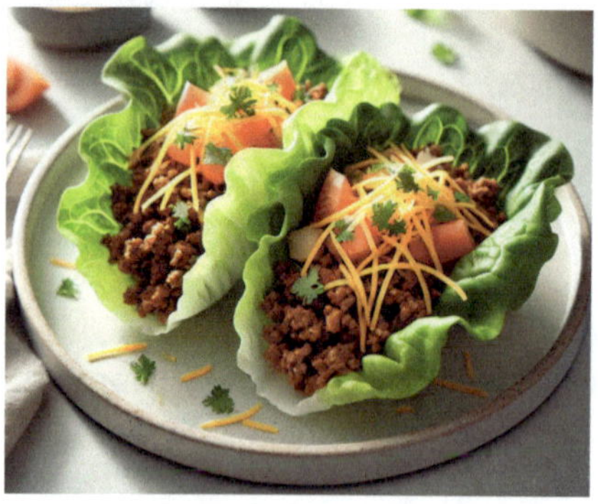

Number of servings: 4

Preparation time: 10 minutes

Cooking time: 15 minutes

Ingredients:

- 1 lb ground beef (85% lean)
- 8 large lettuce leaves (romaine or iceberg)
- 1 tbsp olive oil
- 1 tsp chili powder
- 1/2 tsp cumin
- 1/2 tsp smoked paprika
- 1/2 tsp garlic powder
- Sea salt and black pepper to taste
- 1/2 cup shredded cheddar cheese (optional)
- 1/2 cup diced tomatoes
- 1/4 cup chopped cilantro

Directions:

1. Heat olive oil in a skillet over medium heat. Add the ground beef and cook, breaking it apart, until browned.
2. Stir in chili powder, cumin, smoked paprika, garlic powder, salt, and pepper. Cook for another 2 minutes to combine the flavors.
3. Wash and pat dry the lettuce leaves to use as taco shells.
4. Spoon the beef mixture into the lettuce leaves. Top with cheese, tomatoes, and cilantro.
5. Serve immediately and enjoy.

Nutritional value per serving: Calories: 320, Carbs: 5g, Fiber: 2g, Sugars: 1g, Protein: 26g, Saturated fat: 6g, Unsaturated fat: 10g

Difficulty rating: ★☆☆☆☆

Tips for ingredient variations: Add avocado slices or a dollop of sour cream for extra flavor.

Herb-Crusted Pork Chops with Cauliflower Puree

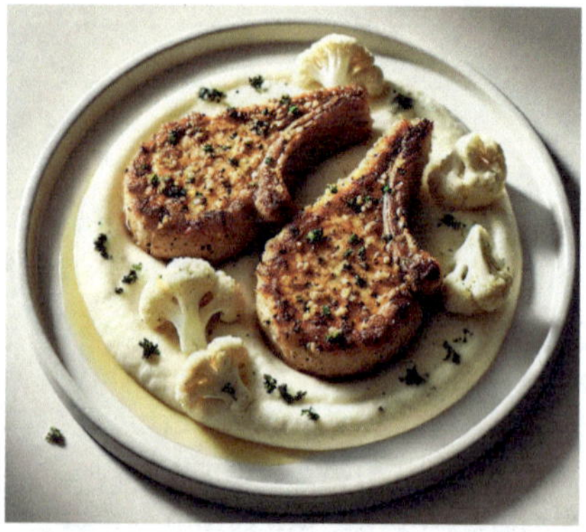

Number of servings: 2

Preparation time: 10 minutes

Cooking time: 20 minutes

Ingredients:

- 2 pork chops (bone-in, about 6 oz each)
- 1 tsp dried rosemary
- 1 tsp dried thyme
- 1 tsp garlic powder
- 1 tbsp olive oil
- 2 cups cauliflower florets
- 1/4 cup heavy cream
- 1 tbsp butter
- Sea salt and black pepper to taste

Directions:

1. Preheat a skillet over medium heat and add olive oil.
2. Rub the pork chops with rosemary, thyme, garlic powder, salt, and pepper.
3. Sear the pork chops for 3-4 minutes on each side, then reduce the heat and cook for an additional 5 minutes or until fully cooked. Remove and rest.
4. Steam the cauliflower florets until tender. Blend with heavy cream, butter, salt, and pepper until smooth.
5. Serve the pork chops over the cauliflower puree.

Nutritional value per serving: Calories: 370, Carbs: 6g, Fiber: 2g, Sugars: 2g, Protein: 30g, Saturated fat: 9g, Unsaturated fat: 8g

Difficulty rating: ★★☆☆☆

Tips for ingredient variations: Add fresh parsley or Parmesan to the cauliflower puree for added depth of flavor.

Roasted Chicken Drumsticks with Zucchini

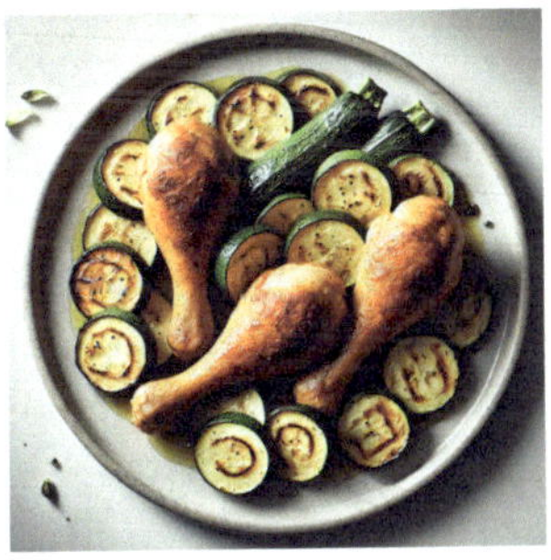

Number of servings: 4

Preparation time: 10 minutes

Cooking time: 40 minutes

Ingredients:

- 8 chicken drumsticks
- 3 medium zucchinis, sliced
- 2 tbsp olive oil
- 2 tsp paprika
- 1 tsp garlic powder
- 1 tsp dried oregano
- Sea salt and black pepper to taste

Directions:

1. Preheat the oven to 375°F (190°C).
2. In a large bowl, toss the drumsticks with 1 tablespoon of olive oil, paprika, garlic powder, oregano, salt, and pepper.
3. Spread the drumsticks on a baking sheet.
4. In the same bowl, toss the zucchini slices with the remaining olive oil, salt, and pepper. Spread them alongside the chicken.
5. Roast for 40 minutes or until the chicken is fully cooked and the zucchini is tender.
6. Serve immediately.

Nutritional value per serving: Calories: 280, Carbs: 4g, Fiber: 1g, Sugars: 2g, Protein: 28g, Saturated fat: 3g, Unsaturated fat: 8g

Difficulty rating: ★☆☆☆☆

Tips for ingredient variations: Sprinkle with Parmesan or drizzle with lemon juice for extra flavor.

Shrimp Scampi with Spaghetti Squash

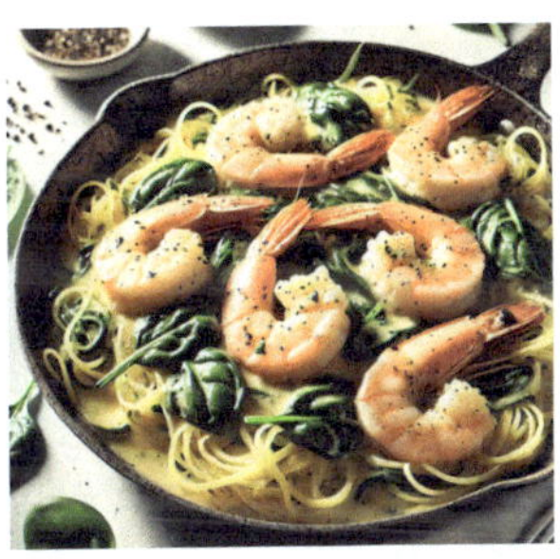

Number of servings: 2

Preparation time: 15 minutes

Cooking time: 25 minutes

Ingredients:

- 1 medium spaghetti squash
- 1 lb shrimp, peeled and deveined
- 3 tbsp butter or ghee
- 3 cloves garlic, minced
- 1/4 cup chicken broth
- 2 tbsp fresh lemon juice
- 2 tbsp chopped parsley
- Sea salt and black pepper to taste
- Red pepper flakes (optional)

Directions:

1. Preheat the oven to 400°F (200°C). After removing the seeds, split the spaghetti squash in half lengthwise and arrange it on a baking sheet cut-side down. Roast for 20-25 minutes until tender.
2. Use a fork to scrape the squash into strands and set aside.
3. In a large skillet, melt the butter over medium heat. Add garlic and sauté for 1-2 minutes until fragrant.
4. Cook the shrimp in the skillet for two to three minutes on each side, or until they are cooked through and pink.
5. Pour in chicken broth and lemon juice, stirring to combine.
6. Toss the spaghetti squash strands into the skillet, mixing well with the shrimp and sauce
7. Season with salt, pepper, and red pepper flakes if desired. Garnish with parsley and serve immediately.

Nutritional value per serving: Calories: 320, Carbs: 10g, Fiber: 4g, Sugars: 4g, Protein: 28g, Saturated fat: 8g, Unsaturated fat: 5g

Difficulty rating: ★★☆☆☆

Tips for ingredient variations: Substitute zucchini noodles for spaghetti squash or add spinach for extra greens.

Keto-Friendly Meatloaf (Almond Flour-Based)

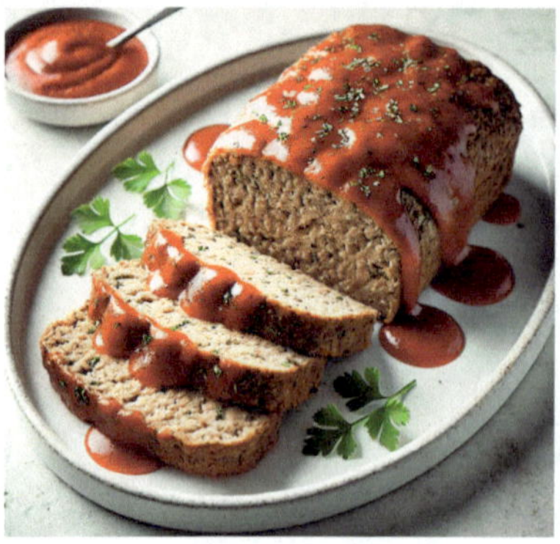

Number of servings: 4

Preparation time: 15 minutes

Cooking time: 50 minutes

Ingredients:

- 1 lb ground beef (grass-fed preferred)
- 1/2 lb ground pork
- 1/2 cup almond flour
- 1 small onion, finely chopped
- 1 egg
- 2 tbsp unsweetened ketchup or tomato paste
- 1 tsp garlic powder
- 1 tsp smoked paprika
- 1 tsp dried oregano
- Sea salt and black pepper to taste

Directions:

1. Preheat the oven to 375°F (190°C). Line a baking dish with parchment paper.
2. In a large bowl, mix ground beef, pork, almond flour, onion, egg, ketchup, garlic powder, paprika, oregano, salt, and pepper until well combined.
3. Shape the mixture into a loaf and place it on the prepared baking dish.
4. Bake for 50 minutes or until the internal temperature reaches 160°F (71°C).
5. Allow the meatloaf to rest for 5 minutes before slicing. Serve warm.

Nutritional value per serving: Calories: 310, Carbs: 5g, Fiber: 2g, Sugars: 1g, Protein: 28g, Saturated fat: 6g, Unsaturated fat: 8g

Difficulty rating: ★★☆☆☆

Tips for ingredient variations: Add grated zucchini or mushrooms to the mix for additional moisture and nutrients.

Grilled Lamb Chops with Spinach Salad

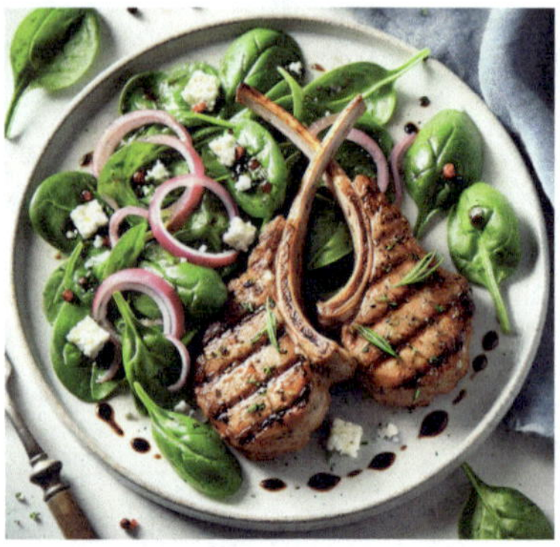

Number of servings: 2

Preparation time: 10 minutes

Cooking time: 15 minutes

Ingredients:

- 4 lamb chops
- 2 tbsp olive oil
- 2 cloves garlic, minced
- 1 tsp dried rosemary
- 4 cups fresh spinach
- 1/2 small red onion, thinly sliced
- 1/4 cup crumbled feta cheese
- 2 tbsp balsamic vinegar
- Sea salt and black pepper to taste

Directions:

1. Rub the lamb chops with olive oil, garlic, rosemary, salt, and pepper. Let marinate for 10 minutes.
2. Preheat a grill or grill pan over medium-high heat. Cook the lamb chops for 3-4 minutes per side for medium-rare or longer for desired doneness.
3. In a large bowl, toss the spinach, red onion, and feta cheese with balsamic vinegar and a drizzle of olive oil.
4. Serve the grilled lamb chops alongside the spinach salad.

Nutritional value per serving: Calories: 420, Carbs: 6g, Fiber: 2g, Sugars: 2g, Protein: 36g, Saturated fat: 10g, Unsaturated fat: 14g

Difficulty rating: ★★☆☆☆

Tips for ingredient variations: Add sliced avocado or roasted walnuts to the salad for additional flavor and texture.

Beef Stroganoff over Cauliflower Rice

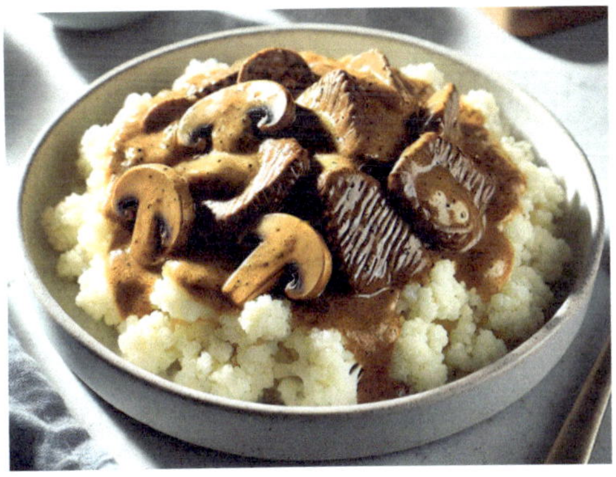

Number of servings: 4

Preparation time: 10 minutes

Cooking time: 20 minutes

Ingredients:

- 1 lb beef sirloin, thinly sliced
- 1 tbsp olive oil
- 1 small onion, chopped
- 2 cups mushrooms, sliced
- 1 cup unsweetened almond milk
- 1/4 cup sour cream
- 1 tbsp Dijon mustard
- 1 tsp paprika
- 4 cups cauliflower rice, steamed
- Sea salt and black pepper to taste

Directions:

1. Heat olive oil in a large skillet over medium heat. Cook the beef slices until browned, then remove and set aside.
2. Add onion and mushrooms to the skillet and sauté until softened.
3. Stir in almond milk, sour cream, Dijon mustard, paprika, salt, and pepper. Simmer for 5 minutes.
4. Return the beef to the skillet and cook for another 5 minutes until heated through.
5. Serve over steamed cauliflower rice.

Nutritional value per serving: Calories: 290, Carbs: 8g, Fiber: 3g, Sugars: 2g, Protein: 26g, Saturated fat: 5g, Unsaturated fat: 6g

Difficulty rating: ★★☆☆☆

Tips for ingredient variations: Use chicken instead of beef or add spinach for extra greens.

Chicken Alfredo with Zoodles

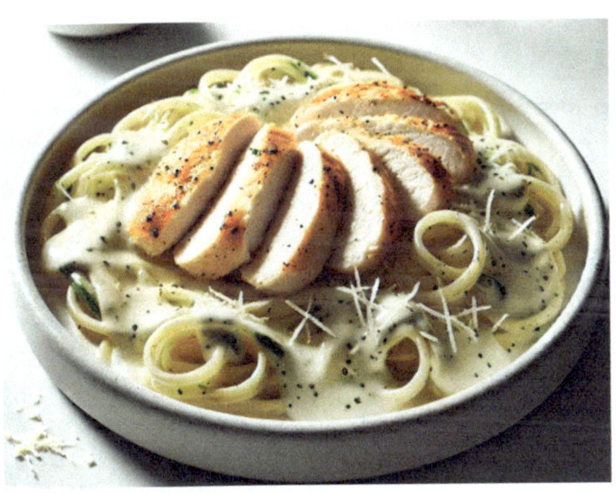

Number of servings: 2

Preparation time: 10 minutes

Cooking time: 15 minutes

Ingredients:

- 2 medium zucchinis, spiralized into zoodles
- 1 lb chicken breast, sliced
- 2 tbsp butter or olive oil
- 1 cup heavy cream
- 1/2 cup grated Parmesan cheese
- 2 cloves garlic, minced
- Sea salt and black pepper to taste

Directions:

1. Heat butter or olive oil in a skillet over medium heat. Cook the chicken slices until golden and cooked through. Remove and set aside.
2. In the same skillet, add garlic and sauté for 1 minute. Pour in heavy cream and simmer for 2 minutes.
3. Stir in Parmesan cheese and season with salt and pepper. Cook until the sauce thickens.
4. Add the chicken and zoodles to the skillet, tossing gently to coat with the sauce.
5. Serve immediately.

Nutritional value per serving: Calories: 340, Carbs: 7g, Fiber: 2g, Sugars: 3g, Protein: 32g, Saturated fat: 10g, Unsaturated fat: 6g

Difficulty rating: ★★☆☆☆

Tips for ingredient variations: Use shrimp instead of chicken or add mushrooms for extra flavor.

Teriyaki Chicken Skewers (Low-Carb Sauce)

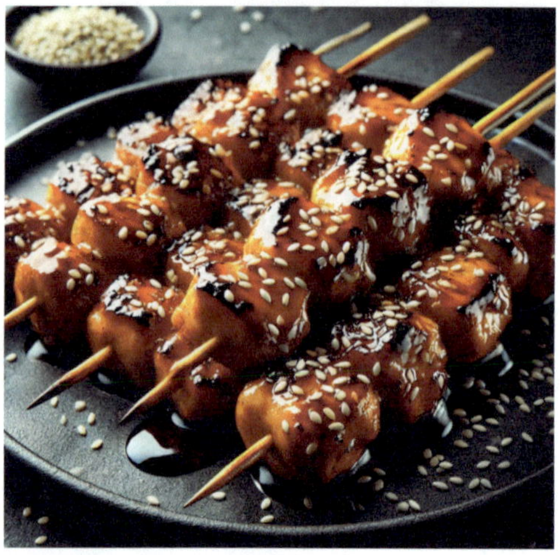

Number of servings: 4

Preparation time: 15 minutes

Cooking time: 15 minutes

Ingredients:

- 1 lb chicken breast, cut into bite-sized pieces
- 1/4 cup soy sauce (low-sodium)
- 2 tbsp coconut aminos
- 1 tbsp sesame oil
- 1 tbsp rice vinegar
- 2 garlic cloves, minced
- 1 tsp grated fresh ginger
- 1 tbsp sesame seeds for garnish
- 1 tbsp green onion, chopped
- 8 bamboo skewers (soaked in water for 30 minutes)

Directions:

1. In a bowl, whisk together soy sauce, coconut aminos, sesame oil, rice vinegar, garlic, and ginger to create the marinade.
2. Let the chicken pieces soak in the marinade for at least fifteen minutes after adding them.
3. Preheat a grill or grill pan over medium-high heat.
4. Put the chicken on skewers and cook it on the grill for 10 to 12 minutes, turning it every so often, until it is cooked through.
5. Sprinkle with sesame seeds and green onion before serving.

Nutritional value per serving: Calories: 180, Carbs: 2g, Fiber: 0g, Sugars: 1g, Protein: 28g, Saturated fat: 1g, Unsaturated fat: 3g

Difficulty rating: ★★☆☆☆

Tips for ingredient variations: Pair with grilled zucchini or cauliflower rice for a complete low-carb meal.

Grilled Halibut with Lemon Dill Sauce

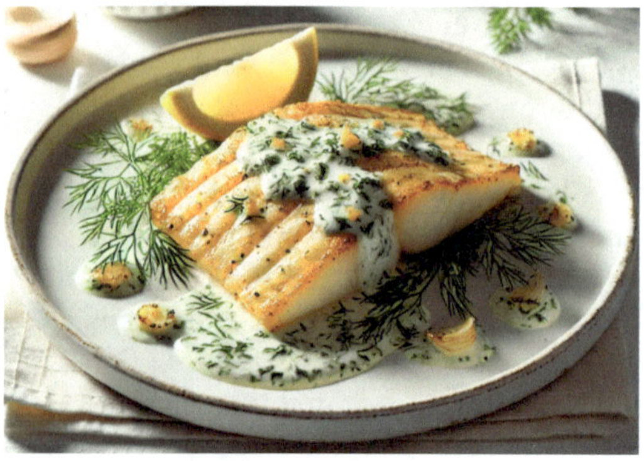

Number of servings: 4

Preparation time: 10 minutes

Cooking time: 12 minutes

Ingredients:

- 4 halibut fillets (6 oz each)
- 2 tbsp olive oil
- 1/4 cup fresh lemon juice
- 2 tbsp fresh dill, chopped
- 1/3 cup plain Greek yogurt
- 1 garlic clove, minced
- Salt and pepper to taste

Directions:

1. Preheat the grill to medium-high heat.
2. Brush the halibut fillets with olive oil and season with salt and pepper.
3. Grill the fillets for 5-6 minutes per side until the fish flakes easily with a fork.
4. In a small bowl, mix lemon juice, dill, yogurt, garlic, and a pinch of salt to create the sauce.
5. Drizzle the sauce over the grilled halibut and serve immediately.

Nutritional value per serving: Calories: 230, Carbs: 3g, Fiber: 0g, Sugars: 1g, Protein: 35g, Saturated fat: 2g, Unsaturated fat: 5g

Difficulty rating: ★☆☆☆☆

Tips for ingredient variations: Replace halibut with cod or salmon if preferred. Add a side of steamed asparagus for a balanced plate.

Turkey and Spinach Stuffed Bell Peppers

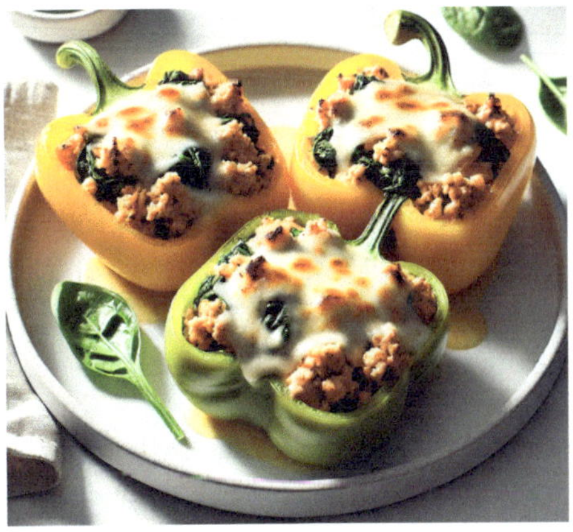

Number of servings: 4

Preparation time: 15 minutes

Cooking time: 30 minutes

Ingredients:

- 4 large bell peppers, halved and seeded
- 1 lb ground turkey
- 1 cup fresh spinach, chopped
- 1/2 cup tomato sauce (low sugar)
- 1/2 cup shredded mozzarella cheese
- 1 tsp Italian seasoning
- 1 tbsp olive oil
- Salt and pepper to taste

Directions:

1. Preheat the oven to 375°F (190°C).
2. Heat olive oil in a skillet over medium heat. Add ground turkey and cook until browned.
3. Stir in spinach, tomato sauce, Italian seasoning, salt, and pepper. Cook for 3-4 minutes.
4. Line a baking sheet with bell pepper halves, then stuff them with the turkey mixture.
5. Sprinkle shredded mozzarella on top of each pepper.
6. Bake for 25-30 minutes until the peppers are tender and the cheese is melted.

Nutritional value per serving: Calories: 210, Carbs: 6g, Fiber: 2g, Sugars: 3g, Protein: 27g, Saturated fat: 4g, Unsaturated fat: 5g

Difficulty rating: ★★☆☆☆

Tips for ingredient variations: Add chopped mushrooms or zucchini to the filling for extra veggies.

Low-Carb Shepherd's Pie (Cauliflower Topping)

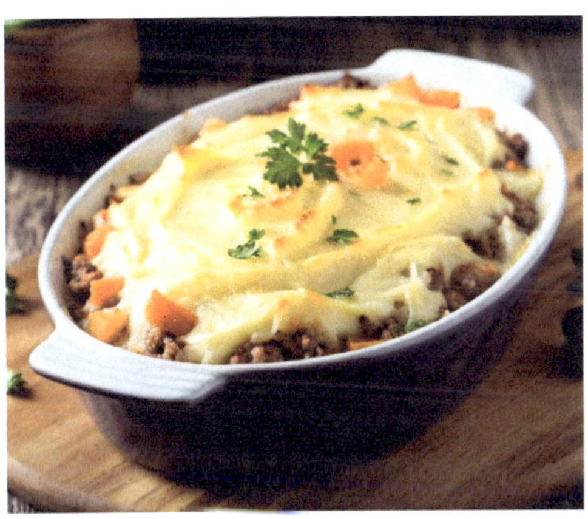

Number of servings: 6

Preparation time: 15 minutes

Cooking time: 30 minutes

Ingredients:

- 1 lb ground beef (grass-fed, lean)
- 1 cup onion, diced
- 1 cup carrots, diced
- 1 cup celery, diced
- 2 cups cauliflower florets
- 1/4 cup heavy cream
- 2 tbsp butter
- 1 tsp garlic powder
- 1 tsp paprika
- Salt and pepper to taste

Directions:

1. Preheat the oven to 400°F (200°C).
2. Boil the cauliflower florets in salted water for 10 minutes until soft. Drain and blend with heavy cream, butter, garlic powder, salt, and pepper until smooth.
3. In a skillet, cook ground beef with onion, carrots, and celery until beef is browned and vegetables are softened. Season with paprika, salt, and pepper.
4. Transfer the beef mixture to a baking dish and spread the cauliflower mash on top.
5. Bake for 20 minutes or until golden on top.

Nutritional value per serving: Calories: 250, Carbs: 8g, Fiber: 3g, Sugars: 3g, Protein: 23g, Saturated fat: 6g, Unsaturated fat: 8g

Difficulty rating: ★★★☆☆

Tips for ingredient variations: Add a handful of grated Parmesan to the cauliflower mash for extra flavor.

Chili Lime Shrimp with Sautéed Peppers

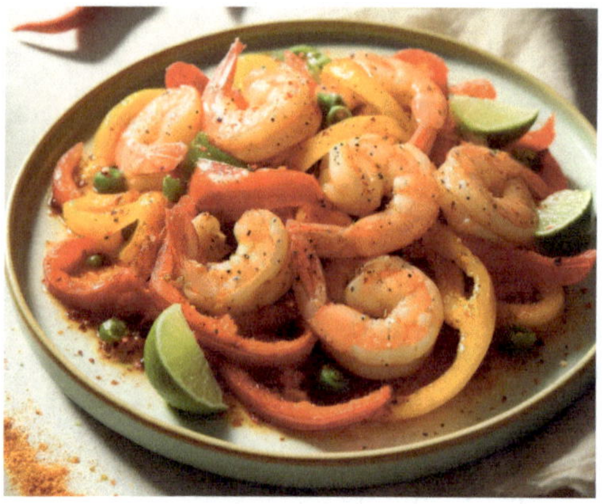

Number of servings: 4

Preparation time: 10 minutes

Cooking time: 10 minutes

Ingredients:

- 1 lb shrimp, peeled and deveined
- 2 bell peppers (red and yellow), sliced
- 2 tbsp olive oil
- 2 tbsp fresh lime juice
- 1 tsp chili powder
- 1 tsp smoked paprika
- 2 garlic cloves, minced
- Salt and pepper to taste

Directions:

1. Toss shrimp with lime juice, chili powder, smoked paprika, garlic, salt, and pepper.
2. Heat 1 tbsp olive oil in a skillet over medium-high heat. Add bell peppers and sauté for 3-4 minutes until tender-crisp. Remove and set aside.
3. Add the remaining olive oil to the skillet and cook the shrimp for 2-3 minutes per side until pink and opaque.
4. Return the peppers to the skillet, toss with the shrimp, and serve warm.

Nutritional value per serving: Calories: 180, Carbs: 5g, Fiber: 2g, Sugars: 2g, Protein: 24g, Saturated fat: 1g, Unsaturated fat: 7g

Difficulty rating: ★★☆☆☆

Tips for ingredient variations: Serve over cauliflower rice or alongside a green salad for a complete meal.

Garlic Parmesan Pork Tenderloin with Roasted Veggies

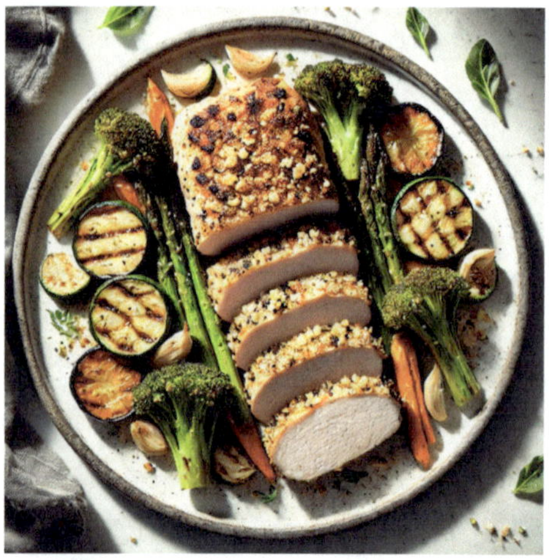

Number of servings: 4

Preparation time: 15 minutes

Cooking time: 30 minutes

Ingredients:

- 1 lb pork tenderloin
- 2 tbsp olive oil
- 2 garlic cloves, minced
- 1/4 cup grated Parmesan cheese
- 1 tsp dried Italian herbs
- 1 cup broccoli florets
- 1 cup zucchini, sliced
- Sea salt and black pepper to taste

Directions:

1. Preheat the oven to 400°F (200°C).
2. Rub the pork tenderloin with olive oil, minced garlic, Parmesan cheese, Italian herbs, salt, and pepper.
3. Place the tenderloin in a baking dish and surround it with broccoli and zucchini. Drizzle vegetables with olive oil and season with salt and pepper.
4. Roast in the oven for 25-30 minutes, or until the pork reaches an internal temperature of 145°F (63°C).
5. Let the pork rest for 5 minutes before slicing. Serve alongside the roasted vegetables.

Nutritional value per serving: Calories: 290, Carbs: 6g, Fiber: 2g, Sugars: 2g, Protein: 28g, Saturated fat: 3g, Unsaturated fat: 9g

Difficulty rating: ★★☆☆☆

Tips for ingredient variations: Swap zucchini for asparagus or add a handful of cherry tomatoes for extra flavor.

Baked Cod with Tomato and Olive Relish

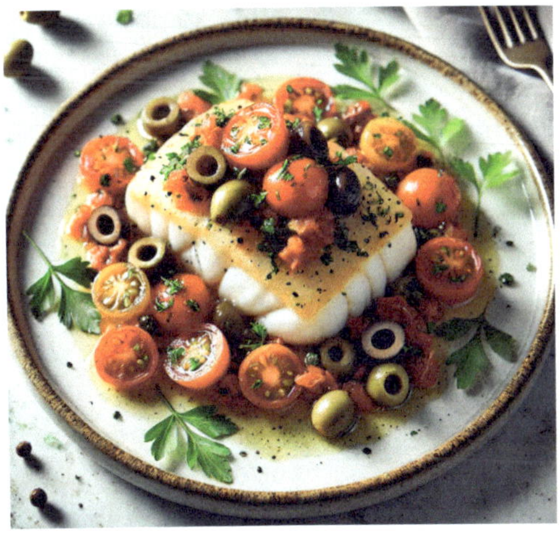

Number of servings: 2

Preparation time: 10 minutes

Cooking time: 15 minutes

Ingredients:

- 2 cod fillets (about 6 oz each)
- 2 tbsp olive oil
- 1/2 cup cherry tomatoes, halved
- 1/4 cup Kalamata olives, sliced
- 1 tbsp capers, drained
- 1 garlic clove, minced
- 1 tbsp fresh parsley, chopped
- Sea salt and black pepper to taste

Directions:

1. Preheat the oven to 375°F (190°C).
2. Drizzle 1 tablespoon of olive oil over the cod fillets in a baking dish. Season with salt and pepper.
3. In a bowl, mix cherry tomatoes, olives, capers, garlic, parsley, and the remaining olive oil.
4. Spoon the tomato and olive mixture over the cod fillets.
5. Bake for 12-15 minutes, or until the cod flakes easily with a fork. Serve warm.

Nutritional value per serving: Calories: 230, Carbs: 5g, Fiber: 1g, Sugars: 2g, Protein: 28g, Saturated fat: 2g, Unsaturated fat: 8g

Difficulty rating: ★☆☆☆☆

Tips for ingredient variations: Add a splash of white wine or lemon juice to the relish for extra depth of flavor.

Chicken Stir-Fry with Sesame Seeds

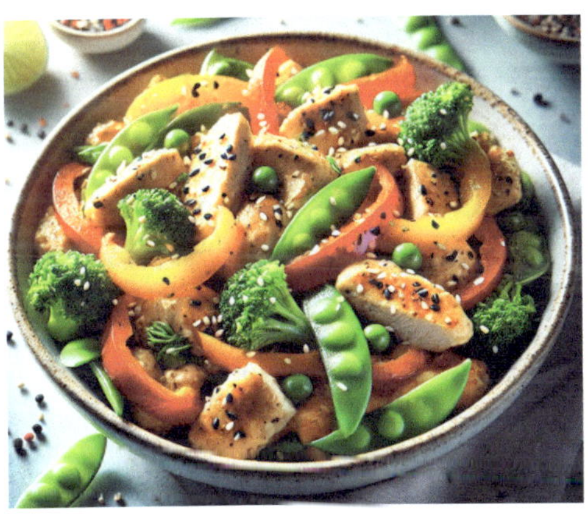

Number of servings: 4

Preparation time: 10 minutes

Cooking time: 15 minutes

Ingredients:

- 1 lb chicken breast, sliced thin
- 2 tbsp sesame oil
- 1 cup bell peppers, sliced
- 1 cup broccoli florets
- 1/2 cup snap peas
- 2 tbsp soy sauce (or tamari for gluten-free)
- 1 tbsp sesame seeds
- 1 garlic clove, minced
- 1 tsp fresh ginger, grated

Directions:

1. In a big skillet or wok, heat the sesame oil over medium-high heat.
2. Add chicken slices and cook until browned, about 5-6 minutes. Remove and set aside.
3. In the same skillet, sauté garlic and ginger for 1 minute. Add bell peppers, broccoli, and snap peas. Stir-fry for 5-6 minutes until tender-crisp.
4. Return the chicken to the skillet, add soy sauce, and toss well to combine. Cook for another 2 minutes.
5. Sprinkle with sesame seeds and serve immediately.

Nutritional value per serving: Calories: 250, Carbs: 7g, Fiber: 2g, Sugars: 3g, Protein: 30g, Saturated fat: 2g, Unsaturated fat: 7g

Difficulty rating: ★☆☆☆☆

Tips for ingredient variations: Add sliced mushrooms or substitute snap peas with zucchini for variety.

Spaghetti Squash Carbonara

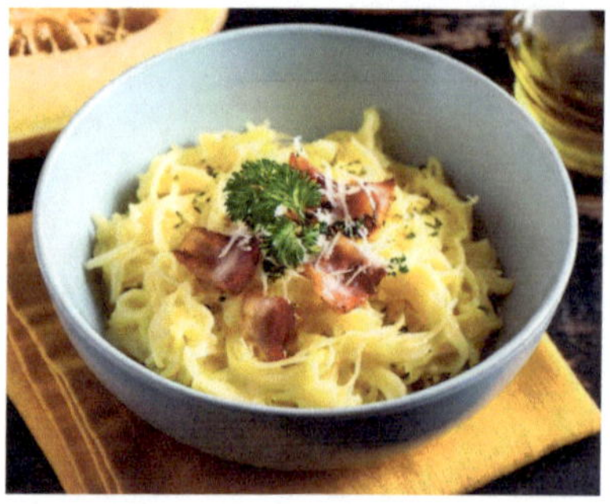

Number of servings: 2

Preparation time: 10 minutes

Cooking time: 40 minutes

Ingredients:

- 1 medium spaghetti squash
- 2 eggs
- 1/4 cup grated Parmesan cheese
- 4 slices cooked bacon, crumbled
- 1 garlic clove, minced
- 1 tbsp olive oil
- Sea salt and black pepper to taste

Directions:

1. Preheat the oven to 400°F (200°C). After removing the seeds, cut the spaghetti squash in half lengthwise. Drizzle with olive oil, season with salt and pepper, and place cut-side down on a baking sheet.
2. Roast till soft, 35 to 40 minutes. Using a fork, scrape the flesh into spaghetti-like pieces.
3. In a bowl, whisk together eggs, Parmesan cheese, and a pinch of black pepper.
4. In a skillet, heat the minced garlic over medium heat. Add the spaghetti squash and toss to coat.
5. Remove from heat, stir in the egg mixture, and mix quickly to create a creamy sauce. Add crumbled bacon and serve.

Nutritional value per serving: Calories: 280, Carbs: 10g, Fiber: 2g, Sugars: 3g, Protein: 18g, Saturated fat: 5g, Unsaturated fat: 7g

Difficulty rating: ★★☆☆☆

Tips for ingredient variations: Add grilled chicken for extra protein or sprinkle with chopped parsley for garnish.

Roasted Duck Breast with Spinach and Mushrooms

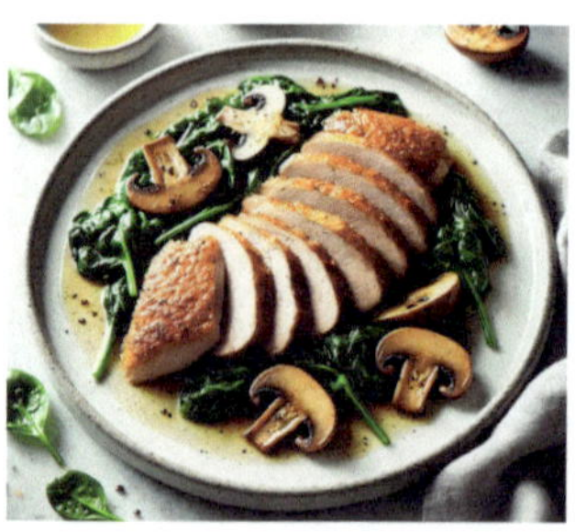

Number of servings: 2

Preparation time: 10 minutes

Cooking time: 25 minutes

Ingredients:

- 2 duck breasts (about 6 oz each)
- 2 cups fresh spinach
- 1 cup mushrooms, sliced
- 2 tbsp olive oil
- 1 garlic clove, minced
- Sea salt and black pepper to taste

Directions:

1. Preheat the oven to 375°F (190°C). Make crosshatch marks on the duck breasts' skin. Add salt and pepper for seasoning.
2. Heat a skillet over medium heat and place the duck breasts skin-side down. Cook for 6-8 minutes to render the fat and crisp the skin. Flip and cook for another 2 minutes.
3. After placing the duck in the oven, roast it for 8 to 10 minutes, or until the internal temperature reaches 135°F (57°C) for medium-rare perfection. Let rest for 5 minutes.
4. In the same skillet, sauté garlic, mushrooms, and spinach in olive oil for 3-4 minutes until tender.
5. Slice the duck and serve over the spinach and mushrooms.

Nutritional value per serving: Calories: 340, Carbs: 4g, Fiber: 1g, Sugars: 1g, Protein: 30g, Saturated fat: 8g, Unsaturated fat: 10g

Difficulty rating: ★★★☆☆

Tips for ingredient variations: Drizzle with balsamic glaze or serve with a side of cauliflower mash for a complete meal.

Broiled Steak with Chimichurri Sauce

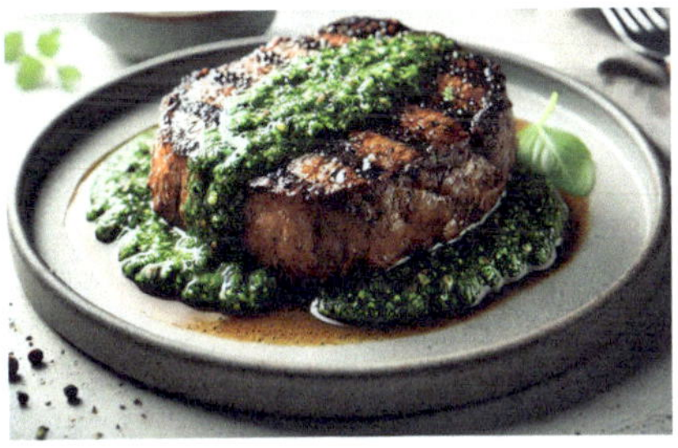

Number of servings: 2

Preparation time: 10 minutes

Cooking time: 8 minutes

Ingredients:

- 2 sirloin steaks (6 oz each)
- 1 tbsp olive oil
- Sea salt and black pepper to taste

For the Chimichurri Sauce:

- 1 cup fresh parsley, chopped
- 1/4 cup fresh cilantro, chopped
- 2 tbsp red wine vinegar
- 3 tbsp olive oil
- 2 garlic cloves, minced
- 1/4 tsp red pepper flakes (optional)
- Sea salt and black pepper to taste

Directions:

1. Put foil on a baking sheet and preheat the broiler.
2. Rub the steaks with olive oil and season with salt and pepper.
3. Place the steaks on the baking sheet and broil for 4-5 minutes per side for medium-rare, or adjust to your preferred doneness.
4. While the steaks cook, prepare the chimichurri sauce by combining all sauce ingredients in a bowl and mixing well.
5. Let the steaks rest for 5 minutes before serving, topped with chimichurri sauce.

Nutritional value per serving: Calories: 380, Carbs: 2g, Fiber: 1g, Sugars: 0g, Protein: 35g, Saturated fat: 5g, Unsaturated fat: 15g

Difficulty rating: ★☆☆☆☆

Tips for ingredient variations: Add a squeeze of fresh lemon to the chimichurri for a citrusy twist or include oregano for an extra herbaceous flavor.

Low-Carb Chicken Parmesan (Almond Flour Breading)

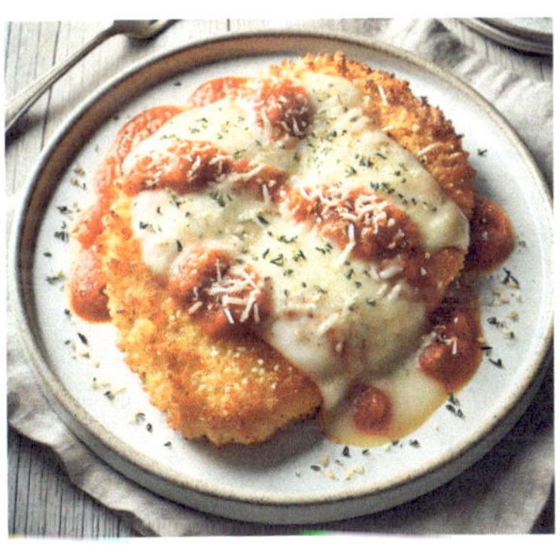

Number of servings: 4

Preparation time: 15 minutes

Cooking time: 25 minutes

Ingredients:

- 4 boneless, skinless chicken breasts
- 1 cup almond flour
- 1/2 cup grated Parmesan cheese
- 1 large egg, beaten
- 1 tsp Italian seasoning
- 1/2 tsp garlic powder
- 1 cup marinara sauce (sugar-free)
- 1 cup shredded mozzarella cheese
- 2 tbsp olive oil

Directions:

1. Preheat the oven to 375°F (190°C).
2. Mix almond flour, Parmesan, Italian seasoning, and garlic powder in a shallow bowl.
3. Before coating each chicken breast with the almond flour mixture, dip it into the beaten egg.
4. Heat olive oil in a large skillet over medium heat. Sear the chicken for 3-4 minutes per side until golden.
5. The chicken should be moved to a baking dish. Add mozzarella cheese and marinara sauce on top of each piece.
6. Bake for 15-20 minutes or until the chicken is cooked through and the cheese is melted.

Nutritional value per serving: Calories: 340, Carbs: 5g, Fiber: 2g, Sugars: 2g, Protein: 40g, Saturated fat: 8g, Unsaturated fat: 12g

Difficulty rating: ★★☆☆☆

Tips for ingredient variations: Add fresh basil or oregano leaves before baking for extra flavor.

Thai Green Curry with Chicken and Zucchini

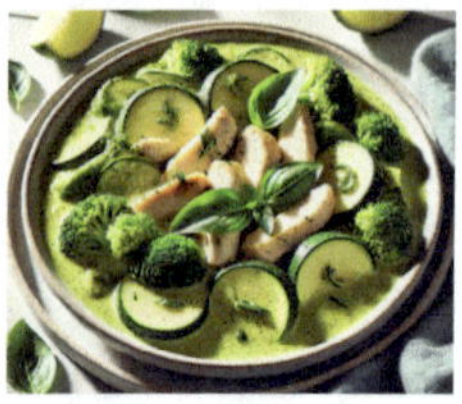

Number of servings: 4
Preparation time: 10 minutes
Cooking time: 20 minutes

Ingredients:

- 1 lb chicken breast, sliced thinly
- 2 medium zucchinis, sliced into half-moons
- 1 tbsp coconut oil
- 2 tbsp green curry paste
- 1 can (13.5 oz) coconut milk (unsweetened)
- 1 cup broccoli florets
- 1/4 cup fresh basil leaves
- 1 tbsp fish sauce (optional)
- Lime wedges for serving

Directions:

1. Heat coconut oil in a large skillet over medium heat. Add the green curry paste and sauté for 1 minute until fragrant.
2. Stir in the coconut milk and bring to a simmer.
3. Add the chicken slices and cook for 5 minutes.
4. Add zucchini and broccoli, cooking for an additional 8-10 minutes until the vegetables are tender and the chicken is fully cooked.
5. Stir in the basil leaves and fish sauce (if using).
6. Serve hot with lime wedges.

Nutritional value per serving: Calories: 290, Carbs: 7g, Fiber: 2g, Sugars: 3g, Protein: 30g, Saturated fat: 12g, Unsaturated fat: 4g

Difficulty rating: ★★☆☆☆

Tips for ingredient variations: Swap chicken for shrimp or tofu for a different protein source.

Grilled Swordfish with Lemon Butter Sauce

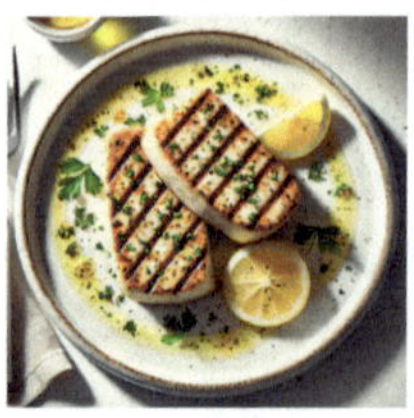

Number of servings: 2
Preparation time: 10 minutes
Cooking time: 10 minutes

Ingredients:

- 2 swordfish steaks (6 oz each)
- 1 tbsp olive oil
- Sea salt and black pepper to taste

For the Lemon Butter Sauce:

- 2 tbsp unsalted butter
- 1 tbsp fresh lemon juice
- 1 tsp lemon zest
- 1 garlic clove, minced
- 1 tbsp fresh parsley, chopped

Directions:

1. Preheat the grill to medium-high heat. Brush swordfish steaks with olive oil and season with salt and pepper.
2. Grill the steaks for 4-5 minutes per side until opaque and cooked through.
3. While the swordfish cooks, melt the butter in a small saucepan over low heat. Stir in the lemon juice, zest, and garlic, cooking for 1-2 minutes.
4. Remove from heat and stir in the parsley.
5. Drizzle the sauce over the grilled swordfish before serving.

Nutritional value per serving: Calories: 300, Carbs: 1g, Fiber: 0g, Sugars: 0g, Protein: 35g, Saturated fat: 7g, Unsaturated fat: 8g

Difficulty rating: ★☆☆☆☆

Tips for ingredient variations: Serve with steamed asparagus or sautéed spinach for a complete meal.

Turkey Burgers with Cauliflower Buns

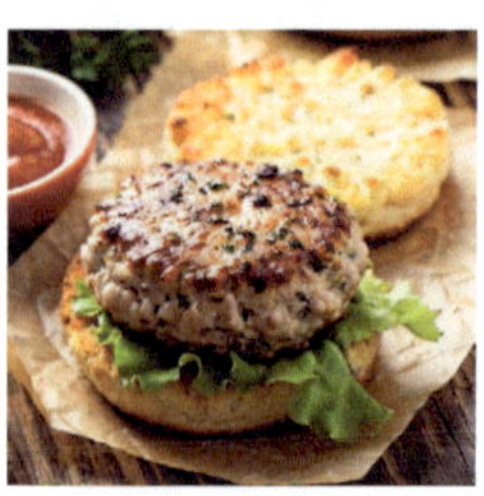

Number of servings: 4
Preparation time: 20 minutes
Cooking time: 15 minutes

Ingredients:

- 1 lb ground turkey
- 1/4 cup grated Parmesan cheese
- 1 garlic clove, minced
- 1 tsp paprika
- 1/2 tsp dried thyme
- Sea salt and black pepper to taste

For the Cauliflower Buns:

- 2 cups riced cauliflower
- 1 egg, beaten
- 1/4 cup shredded mozzarella cheese
- 1/4 tsp garlic powder

Directions:

1. Preheat the oven to 400°F (200°C) and line a baking sheet with parchment paper.
2. Mix riced cauliflower, egg, mozzarella, and garlic powder in a bowl. Form into 8 small circles and bake for 12-15 minutes until firm and golden.
3. In another bowl, combine turkey, Parmesan, garlic, paprika, thyme, salt, and pepper. Form into 4 patties.
4. Cook the patties in a skillet over medium heat for 5-6 minutes per side, or until fully cooked.
5. Assemble the burgers using the cauliflower buns and your choice of toppings, such as lettuce, tomato, or avocado.

Nutritional value per serving: Calories: 280, Carbs: 6g, Fiber: 2g, Sugars: 1g, Protein: 30g, Saturated fat: 5g, Unsaturated fat: 7g

Difficulty rating: ★★☆☆☆

Tips for ingredient variations: Add slices of cheddar or a dollop of guacamole for added flavor.

Main Vegetarian

Cauliflower Mac and Cheese

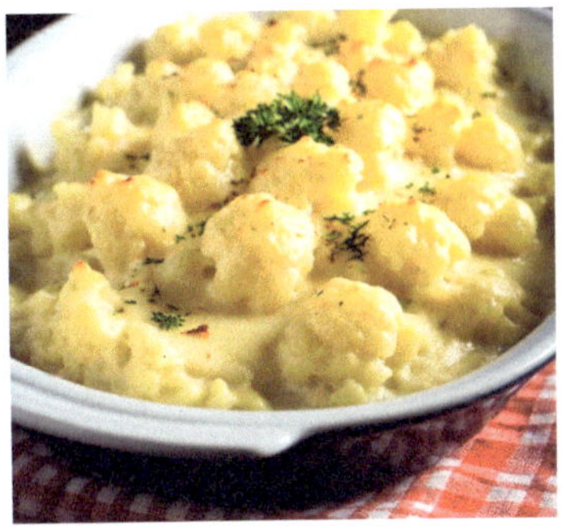

Number of servings: 4

Preparation time: 10 minutes

Cooking time: 20 minutes

Ingredients:

- 1 medium head cauliflower, cut into florets
- 1 1/2 cups shredded cheddar cheese
- 1/2 cup heavy cream
- 1/4 cup grated Parmesan cheese
- 1 tbsp cream cheese
- 1/2 tsp garlic powder
- 1/4 tsp paprika
- Sea salt and black pepper to taste

Directions:

1. Preheat the oven to 375°F (190°C).
2. Steam or boil the cauliflower florets until tender, about 8-10 minutes. Drain and set aside.
3. In a saucepan over medium heat, combine heavy cream, cream cheese, and garlic powder. Stir until smooth.
4. Gradually add cheddar and Parmesan cheese, stirring until melted and combined. Season with paprika, salt, and pepper.
5. Mix the cauliflower into the cheese sauce until well coated. Transfer to a baking dish.
6. Bake for 10 minutes, or until the top is golden and bubbly. Serve hot.

Nutritional value per serving: Calories: 210, Carbs: 6g, Fiber: 3g, Sugars: 2g, Protein: 12g, Saturated fat: 9g, Unsaturated fat: 3g

Difficulty rating: ★☆☆☆☆

Tips for ingredient variations: Sprinkle crumbled bacon or add chopped chives for extra flavor.

Eggplant Lasagna with Ricotta and Spinach

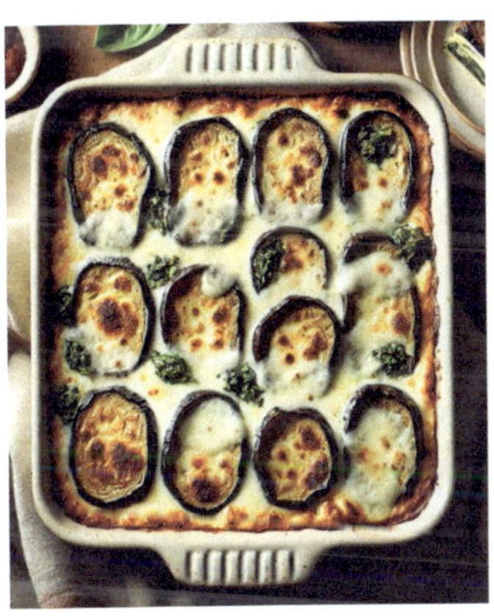

Number of servings: 6

Preparation time: 20 minutes

Cooking time: 40 minutes

Ingredients:

- 2 medium eggplants, sliced lengthwise into 1/4-inch slices
- 2 cups ricotta cheese
- 1 cup shredded mozzarella cheese
- 1/2 cup grated Parmesan cheese
- 2 cups fresh spinach, chopped
- 2 cups marinara sauce (sugar-free)
- 1 egg
- 1 tsp dried Italian herbs
- Sea salt and black pepper to taste

Directions:

1. Preheat the oven to 375°F (190°C). Lightly salt the eggplant slices and let them sit for 10 minutes to remove excess moisture. Pat dry.
2. In a bowl, mix ricotta, spinach, egg, Parmesan, Italian herbs, salt, and pepper until well combined.
3. In a baking dish, spread a thin layer of marinara sauce. Layer eggplant slices, ricotta mixture, marinara sauce, and mozzarella cheese. Repeat until all ingredients are used, finishing with a layer of mozzarella.
4. Cover with foil and bake for 30 minutes. Remove foil and bake for an additional 10 minutes, or until the top is golden and bubbly.
5. Let cool for 5 minutes before serving.

Nutritional value per serving: Calories: 250, Carbs: 8g, Fiber: 3g, Sugars: 4g, Protein: 14g, Saturated fat: 8g, Unsaturated fat: 2g

Difficulty rating: ★★☆☆☆

Tips for ingredient variations: Add ground turkey or beef for an extra protein boost.

Zucchini Fritters with Sour Cream Dip

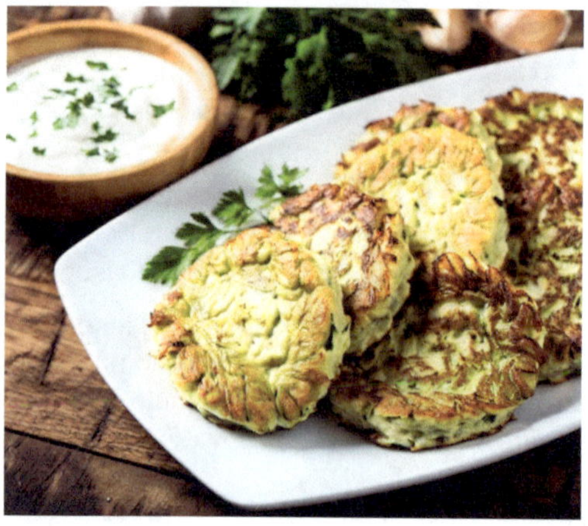

Number of servings: 4

Preparation time: 10 minutes

Cooking time: 15 minutes

Ingredients:

- 2 medium zucchinis, grated and squeezed to remove excess moisture
- 2 eggs
- 1/4 cup almond flour
- 1/4 cup grated Parmesan cheese
- 1/2 tsp garlic powder
- Sea salt and black pepper to taste
- 1 tbsp olive oil or butter for frying
- 1/2 cup sour cream (for dipping)

Directions:

1. In a bowl, mix grated zucchini, eggs, almond flour, Parmesan, garlic powder, salt, and pepper until well combined.
2. Heat olive oil or butter in a skillet over medium heat.
3. Scoop 2-3 tablespoons of the mixture for each fritter and flatten slightly in the pan.
4. Cook for 3-4 minutes on each side, or until golden brown.
5. Serve warm with sour cream dip on the side.

Nutritional value per serving: Calories: 150, Carbs: 4g, Fiber: 1g, Sugars: 2g, Protein: 7g, Saturated fat: 3g, Unsaturated fat: 5g

Difficulty rating: ★☆☆☆☆

Tips for ingredient variations: Add chopped scallions or dill to the fritter mixture for extra flavor.

Grilled Portobello Mushrooms with Goat Cheese

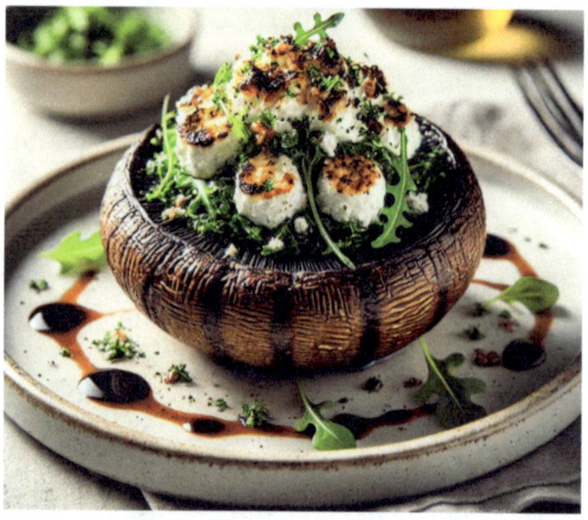

Number of servings: 2

Preparation time: 10 minutes

Cooking time: 10 minutes

Ingredients:

- 4 large Portobello mushrooms, stems removed
- 1/3 cup goat cheese, crumbled
- 1 tbsp olive oil
- 1 garlic clove, minced
- 1 tbsp fresh parsley, chopped
- Sea salt and black pepper to taste

Directions:

1. Preheat grill or grill pan to medium-high heat.
2. Brush the mushrooms with olive oil and season with salt, pepper, and minced garlic.
3. Grill the mushrooms for 4-5 minutes per side, or until tender.
4. Top each mushroom with crumbled goat cheese and cook for an additional 2 minutes, allowing the cheese to soften.
5. Garnish with fresh parsley and serve immediately.

Nutritional value per serving: Calories: 140, Carbs: 5g, Fiber: 2g, Sugars: 2g, Protein: 7g, Saturated fat: 4g, Unsaturated fat: 5g

Difficulty rating: ★☆☆☆☆

Tips for ingredient variations: Add a drizzle of balsamic glaze for a touch of sweetness.

Broccoli and Tofu Stir-Fry with Almond Butter Sauce

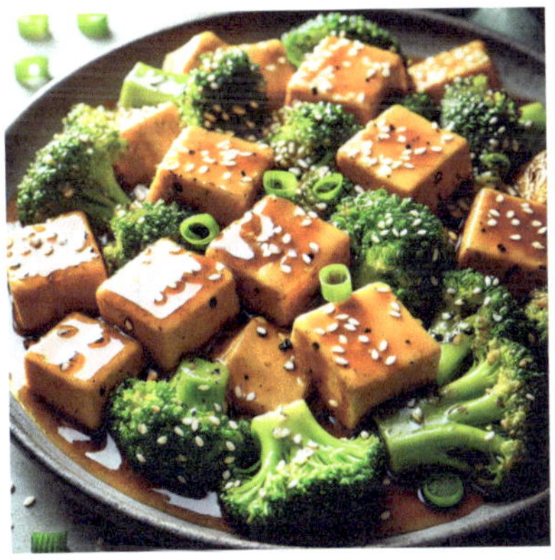

Number of servings: 3

Preparation time: 10 minutes

Cooking time: 15 minutes

Ingredients:

- 2 cups broccoli florets
- 1 block (200g) firm tofu, cubed
- 2 tbsp almond butter
- 2 tbsp soy sauce or tamari
- 1 tbsp sesame oil
- 1 garlic clove, minced
- 1 tsp ginger, grated
- 1/4 tsp red pepper flakes (optional)
- 1 tbsp sesame seeds for garnish

Directions:

1. Heat sesame oil in a skillet over medium heat. Add tofu cubes and cook until golden on all sides, about 5-7 minutes. Remove and set aside.
2. In the same skillet, sauté broccoli florets until tender but crisp, about 5 minutes.
3. In a small bowl, whisk together almond butter, soy sauce, garlic, ginger, and red pepper flakes. Add a splash of water to thin if needed.
4. Return tofu to the skillet, pour the almond butter sauce over, and toss to coat evenly. Cook for 2 minutes to warm through.
5. Garnish with sesame seeds and serve.

Nutritional value per serving: Calories: 210, Carbs: 7g, Fiber: 3g, Sugars: 2g, Protein: 12g, Saturated fat: 2g, Unsaturated fat: 7g

Difficulty rating: ★★☆☆☆

Tips for ingredient variations: Add sliced bell peppers or snap peas for more color and crunch.

Spinach and Ricotta Stuffed Peppers

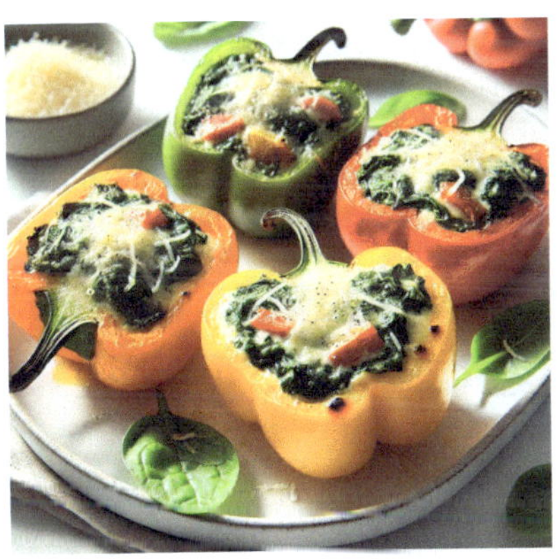

Number of servings: 4

Preparation time: 15 minutes

Cooking time: 25 minutes

Ingredients:

- 4 medium bell peppers (any color), halved and seeded
- 1 cup fresh spinach, chopped
- 1 cup ricotta cheese
- 1/3 cup grated Parmesan cheese
- 1/2 tsp garlic powder
- 1/2 tsp Italian seasoning
- 1 tbsp olive oil
- Sea salt and black pepper to taste

Directions:

1. Preheat the oven to 375°F (190°C).
2. Place the halved peppers on a baking dish, drizzle with olive oil, and sprinkle with a pinch of salt and pepper. Roast for 10 minutes.
3. While the peppers roast, mix ricotta, spinach, Parmesan, garlic powder, Italian seasoning, salt, and pepper in a bowl.
4. After taking the peppers out of the oven, stuff the ricotta mixture into each half.
5. Return to the oven and bake for 15 minutes or until the filling is heated through and the tops are slightly golden.
6. Serve warm and enjoy.

Nutritional value per serving: Calories: 180, Carbs: 6g, Fiber: 2g, Sugars: 3g, Protein: 10g, Saturated fat: 6g, Unsaturated fat: 3g

Difficulty rating: ★☆☆☆☆

Tips for ingredient variations: Add cooked ground turkey or shredded chicken for extra protein.

Broccoli Cheddar Soup (Low-Carb Version)

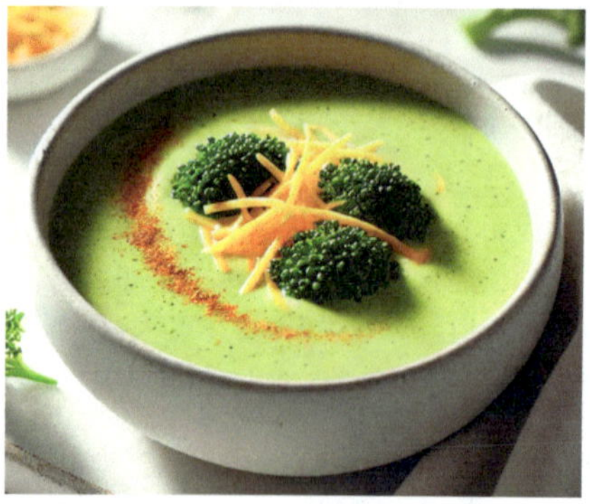

Number of servings: 4

Preparation time: 10 minutes

Cooking time: 20 minutes

Ingredients:

- 4 cups broccoli florets
- 1 tbsp butter
- 1 small onion, diced
- 2 garlic cloves, minced
- 3 cups unsweetened almond milk or chicken broth
- 1 cup shredded cheddar cheese
- 1/2 cup heavy cream
- 1/2 tsp smoked paprika
- Sea salt and black pepper to taste

Directions:

1. Heat the butter in a large pot over medium heat. Add the onion and garlic and sauté until softened, about 3 minutes.
2. Add the broccoli florets and cook for 5 minutes.
3. Pour in the almond milk or chicken broth, season with smoked paprika, salt, and pepper, and bring to a simmer. Cook for 10 minutes or until the broccoli is tender.
4. Use an immersion blender to puree the soup to your desired consistency.
5. Stir in the cheddar cheese and heavy cream until melted and well combined.
6. Serve hot and garnish with extra cheddar or a sprinkle of paprika.

Nutritional value per serving: Calories: 240, Carbs: 7g, Fiber: 3g, Sugars: 2g, Protein: 12g, Saturated fat: 9g, Unsaturated fat: 3g

Difficulty rating: ★★☆☆☆

Tips for ingredient variations: Top with crispy bacon bits for added flavor and crunch.

Cauliflower Crust Pizza with Mozzarella

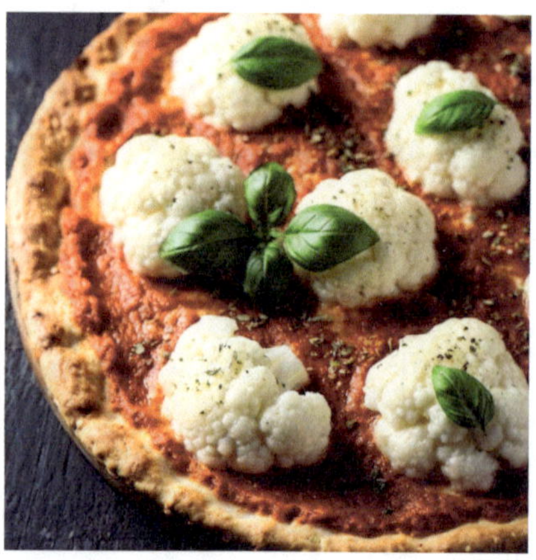

Number of servings: 2

Preparation time: 20 minutes

Cooking time: 25 minutes

Ingredients:

- 1 medium cauliflower head, riced (about 2 cups)
- 1/2 cup shredded mozzarella cheese
- 1/4 cup grated Parmesan cheese
- 1 large egg
- 1 tsp Italian seasoning
- 1/4 cup marinara sauce (low-sugar)
- 1/2 cup shredded mozzarella cheese (for topping)
- Favorite toppings (pepperoni, mushrooms, bell peppers)

Directions:

1. Preheat the oven to 400°F (200°C) and line a baking sheet with parchment paper.
2. Steam the riced cauliflower until tender, about 5 minutes. Let cool, then squeeze out excess water using a clean kitchen towel.
3. In a bowl, mix the cauliflower with mozzarella, Parmesan, egg, and Italian seasoning until well combined.
4. Press the mixture onto the prepared baking sheet to form a pizza crust. Bake for 15 minutes or until golden brown.
5. Remove the crust from the oven, spread marinara sauce over the top, and sprinkle with mozzarella and your chosen toppings.
6. Bake for ten more minutes, or until the cheese is bubbling and melted.
7. Slice and serve hot.

Nutritional value per serving: Calories: 250, Carbs: 8g, Fiber: 3g, Sugars: 3g, Protein: 18g, Saturated fat: 8g, Unsaturated fat: 3g

Difficulty rating: ★★☆☆☆

Tips for ingredient variations: Use pesto instead of marinara for a different flavor profile.

Greek Salad with Grilled Halloumi Cheese

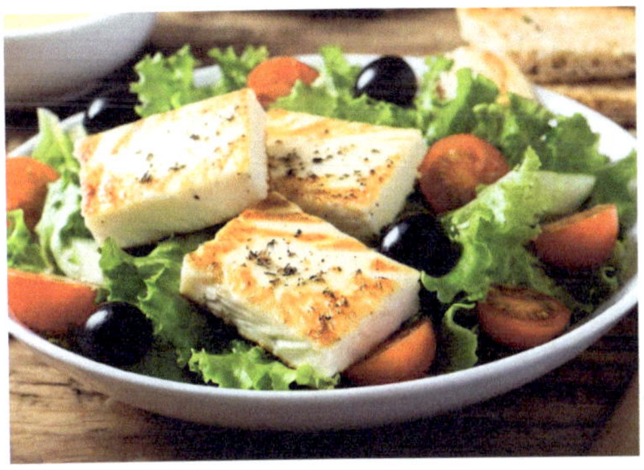

Number of servings: 2

Preparation time: 10 minutes

Cooking time: 5 minutes

Ingredients:

- 1 block of halloumi cheese (about 200g), sliced
- 2 cups mixed greens
- 1/2 cucumber, sliced
- 1/4 cup cherry tomatoes, halved
- 1/4 cup kalamata olives
- 2 tbsp olive oil
- 1 tbsp red wine vinegar
- 1 tsp dried oregano
- Sea salt and black pepper to taste

Directions:

1. Heat a non-stick skillet over medium-high heat and grill the halloumi slices for 1-2 minutes on each side until golden brown.
2. In a large bowl, combine the mixed greens, cucumber, cherry tomatoes, and olives.
3. In a small bowl, whisk together olive oil, red wine vinegar, oregano, salt, and pepper to create the dressing.
4. Add the grilled halloumi to the salad and drizzle with the dressing.
5. Toss gently and serve immediately.

Nutritional value per serving: Calories: 320, Carbs: 6g, Fiber: 2g, Sugars: 2g, Protein: 18g, Saturated fat: 10g, Unsaturated fat: 8g

Difficulty rating: ★☆☆☆☆

Tips for ingredient variations: Add sliced avocado for extra creaminess or sprinkle with roasted sunflower seeds for crunch.

Creamy Mushroom and Spinach Casserole

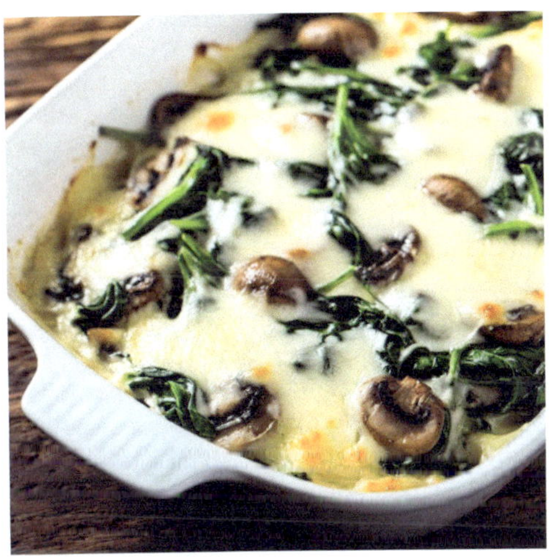

Number of servings: 4

Preparation time: 10 minutes

Cooking time: 25 minutes

Ingredients:

- 2 cups fresh spinach
- 2 cups mushrooms, sliced
- 1 cup heavy cream
- 1/2 cup grated Parmesan cheese
- 1/2 cup shredded mozzarella cheese
- 1 garlic clove, minced
- 1 tbsp olive oil
- Sea salt and black pepper to taste

Directions:

1. Preheat the oven to 375°F (190°C).
2. Heat olive oil in a skillet over medium heat. Add garlic and mushrooms, cooking for 5 minutes until softened.
3. Add spinach to the skillet and cook until wilted, about 2 minutes. Season with salt and pepper.
4. Transfer the mixture to a casserole dish. Pour heavy cream over the top, then sprinkle with Parmesan and mozzarella.
5. Bake for 15-20 minutes or until bubbly and golden.
6. Serve hot as a side or main dish.

Nutritional value per serving: Calories: 270, Carbs: 5g, Fiber: 2g, Sugars: 2g, Protein: 12g, Saturated fat: 12g, Unsaturated fat: 3g

Difficulty rating: ★★☆☆☆

Tips for ingredient variations: Add cooked chicken or turkey for a heartier meal.

Roasted Cauliflower Soup with Thyme

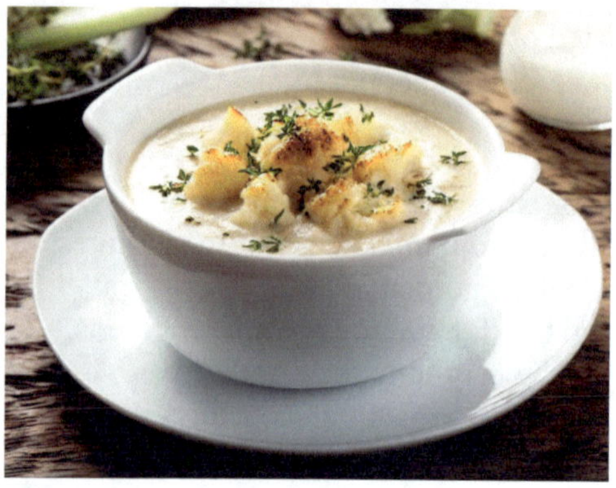

Number of servings: 4

Preparation time: 10 minutes

Cooking time: 30 minutes

Ingredients:

- 1 medium head of cauliflower, chopped into florets
- 1 medium onion, diced
- 2 garlic cloves, minced
- 3 cups vegetable or chicken broth
- 1 cup unsweetened almond milk
- 1 tbsp olive oil
- 1 tsp dried thyme
- Salt and black pepper to taste
- Fresh thyme leaves for garnish

Directions:

1. Preheat the oven to 400°F (200°C). Toss the cauliflower florets with olive oil, salt, and pepper, and spread them on a baking sheet. Roast for 20-25 minutes until golden and tender.
2. In a large pot, sauté the onion and garlic over medium heat until softened, about 3-5 minutes.
3. Add the roasted cauliflower, broth, almond milk, and dried thyme to the pot. Bring to a simmer and cook for 5-10 minutes.
4. Use an immersion blender to puree the soup until smooth. Adjust seasoning with salt and pepper.
5. Serve hot, garnished with fresh thyme leaves.

Nutritional value per serving: Calories: 120, Carbs: 8g, Fiber: 3g, Sugars: 2g, Protein: 4g, Saturated fat: 1g, Unsaturated fat: 3g

Difficulty rating: ★☆☆☆☆

Tips for ingredient variations: Add a dollop of Greek yogurt for extra creaminess or sprinkle with roasted pumpkin seeds for texture.

Shakshuka with Spinach and Feta

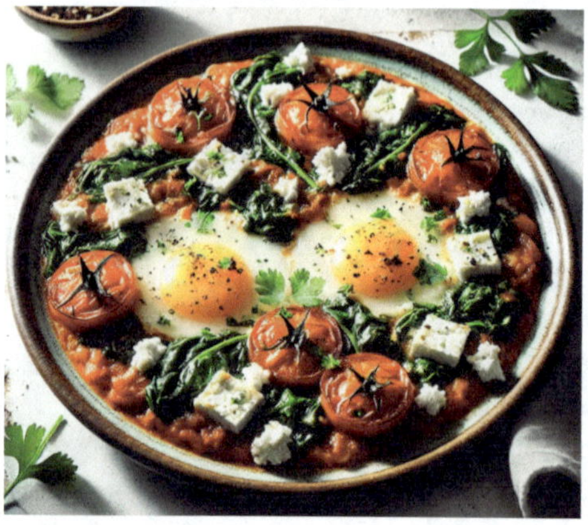

Number of servings: 2

Preparation time: 10 minutes

Cooking time: 15 minutes

Ingredients:

- 1 tbsp olive oil
- 1 small onion, diced
- 1 red bell pepper, diced
- 2 cups fresh spinach, chopped
- 3 garlic cloves, minced
- 1 can (14 oz) diced tomatoes
- 1 tsp ground cumin
- 1 tsp smoked paprika
- 4 large eggs
- 1/3 cup crumbled feta cheese
- Salt and black pepper to taste
- Fresh parsley for garnish

Directions:

1. Heat the olive oil in a large skillet over medium heat. Add the onion and bell pepper, cooking until softened, about 5 minutes.
2. Stir in the garlic, cumin, and smoked paprika, cooking for 1 minute until fragrant.
3. Add the diced tomatoes and spinach. Simmer for 5 minutes, stirring occasionally.
4. Make small wells in the tomato mixture and crack an egg into each. Cover the skillet and cook until the egg whites are set, about 5 minutes.
5. Sprinkle with feta cheese and garnish with fresh parsley. Serve immediately.

Nutritional value per serving: Calories: 230, Carbs: 10g, Fiber: 4g, Sugars: 6g, Protein: 14g, Saturated fat: 6g, Unsaturated fat: 5g

Difficulty rating: ★★☆☆☆

Tips for ingredient variations: Add diced zucchini or mushrooms for extra vegetables. Adjust spices for a spicier dish.

Kale Salad with Avocado and Pumpkin Seeds

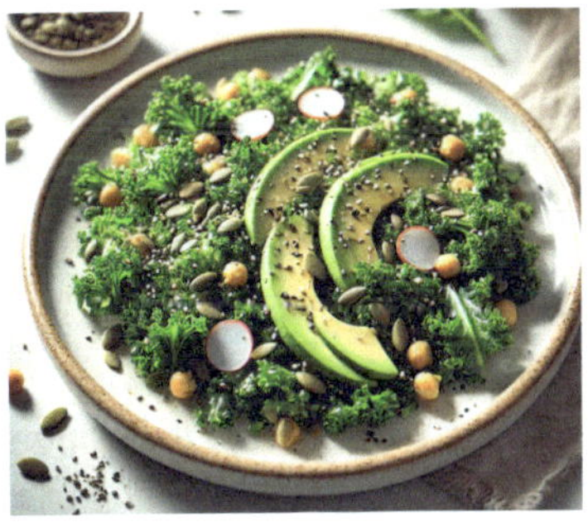

Number of servings: 2
Preparation time: 10 minutes
Cooking time: 0 minutes

Ingredients:

- 4 cups kale, chopped and massaged
- 1 avocado, diced
- 1/4 cup pumpkin seeds
- 1 tbsp lemon juice
- 1 tbsp olive oil
- Salt and black pepper to taste

Directions:

1. Place the chopped kale in a large bowl. Drizzle with olive oil and massage with your hands until the leaves are tender.
2. Add the diced avocado and pumpkin seeds to the bowl.
3. Drizzle with lemon juice, sprinkle with salt and pepper, and toss gently to combine.
4. Serve immediately as a refreshing side dish or light lunch.

Nutritional value per serving: Calories: 190, Carbs: 7g, Fiber: 4g, Sugars: 1g, Protein: 5g, Saturated fat: 2g, Unsaturated fat: 14g

Difficulty rating: ★☆☆☆☆

Tips for ingredient variations: Top with grilled chicken or boiled eggs for added protein.

Roasted Brussels Sprouts with Balsamic Glaze

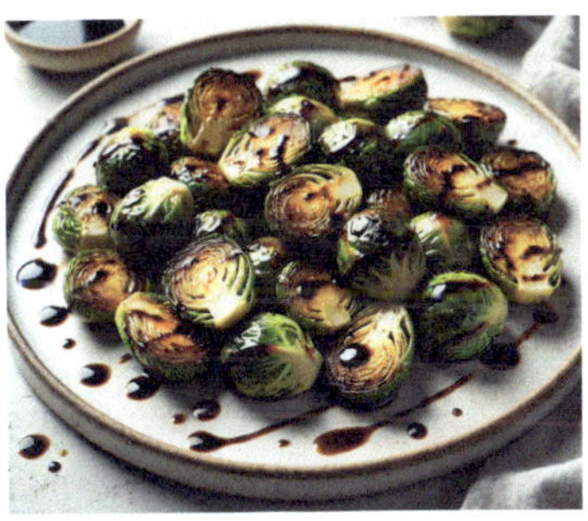

Number of servings: 4
Preparation time: 5 minutes
Cooking time: 20 minutes

Ingredients:

- 1 lb Brussels sprouts, halved
- 1 tbsp olive oil
- 2 tbsp balsamic vinegar
- 1 tsp honey or sugar-free sweetener
- Salt and black pepper to taste

Directions:

1. Preheat the oven to 400°F (200°C). Season the Brussels sprouts with salt, pepper, and olive oil before spreading them out on a baking pan.
2. Roast for 15-20 minutes until golden and tender.
3. In a small saucepan, heat the balsamic vinegar and honey until slightly thickened, about 2-3 minutes.
4. Drizzle the balsamic glaze over the roasted Brussels sprouts and toss to coat. Serve hot.

Nutritional value per serving: Calories: 110, Carbs: 9g, Fiber: 4g, Sugars: 3g, Protein: 3g, Saturated fat: 1g, Unsaturated fat: 5g

Difficulty rating: ★☆☆☆☆

Tips for ingredient variations: Sprinkle with Parmesan cheese or crispy bacon bits for added flavor.

Cucumber Noodles with Peanut Sauce

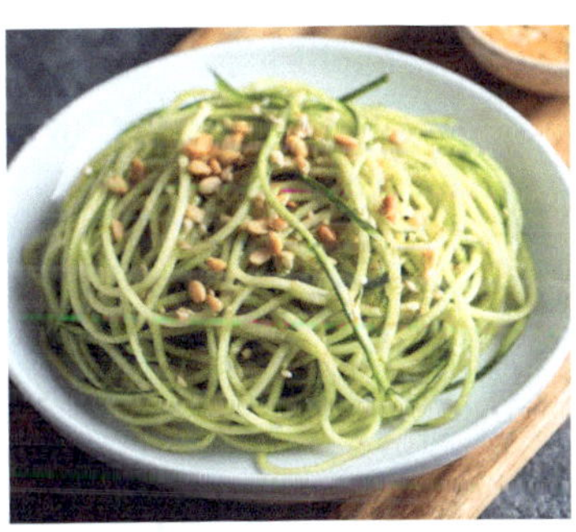

Number of servings: 2
Preparation time: 10 minutes
Cooking time: 0 minutes

Ingredients:

- 2 large cucumbers, spiralized into noodles
- 2 tbsp natural peanut butter
- 1 tbsp soy sauce (or coconut aminos)
- 1 tbsp rice vinegar
- 1 tsp sesame oil
- 1/4 tsp chili flakes (optional)
- 1 tbsp chopped peanuts for garnish
- 1 tbsp chopped cilantro for garnish

Directions:

1. Spiralize the cucumbers into noodles and place them in a large bowl.
2. In a small bowl, whisk together peanut butter, soy sauce, rice vinegar, sesame oil, and chili flakes until smooth.
3. Pour the peanut sauce over the cucumber noodles and toss gently to coat.
4. Garnish with chopped peanuts and cilantro before serving.

Nutritional value per serving: Calories: 160, Carbs: 8g, Fiber: 2g, Sugars: 3g, Protein: 6g, Saturated fat: 2g, Unsaturated fat: 8g

Difficulty rating: ★☆☆☆☆

Tips for ingredient variations: Add grilled shrimp or shredded chicken for a more filling meal.

Sides

Roasted Cauliflower with Garlic and Parmesan

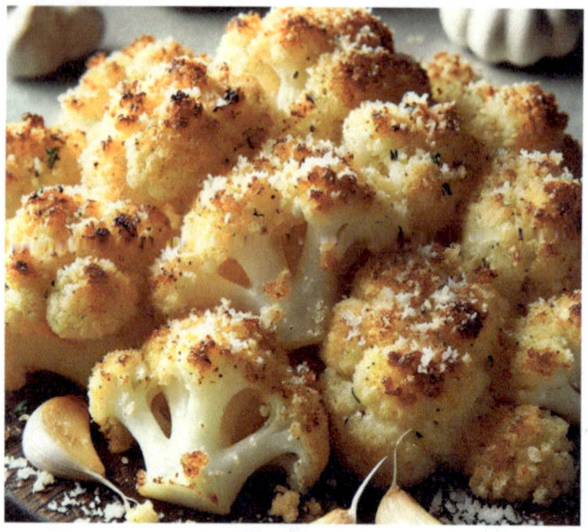

Number of servings: 4

Preparation time: 10 minutes

Cooking time: 25 minutes

Ingredients:

- 1 medium head of cauliflower, cut into florets
- 3 tbsp olive oil
- 3 garlic cloves, minced
- 1/3 cup grated Parmesan cheese
- 1 tsp dried oregano
- Sea salt and black pepper to taste

Directions:

1. Preheat the oven to 400°F (200°C).
2. In a large mixing bowl, toss the cauliflower florets with olive oil, garlic, oregano, salt, and pepper until well coated.
3. Spread the cauliflower evenly on a baking sheet lined with parchment paper.
4. Roast in the oven for 20 minutes, stirring halfway through.
5. After adding the Parmesan cheese to the cauliflower, put it back in the oven for five more minutes, or until it has melted and turned a light golden color.
6. Serve warm as a side dish.

Nutritional value per serving: Calories: 140, Carbs: 7g, Fiber: 3g, Sugars: 2g, Protein: 6g, Saturated fat: 2g, Unsaturated fat: 5g

Difficulty rating: ★☆☆☆☆

Tips for ingredient variations: Add a pinch of red pepper flakes for a hint of heat, or substitute Parmesan with Pecorino for a stronger flavor.

Sautéed Spinach with Olive Oil and Garlic

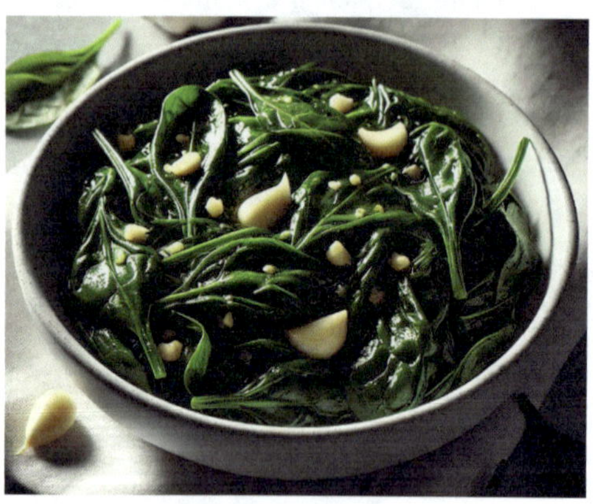

Number of servings: 2

Preparation time: 5 minutes

Cooking time: 5 minutes

Ingredients:

- 6 cups fresh spinach, washed and drained
- 2 tbsp olive oil
- 3 garlic cloves, thinly sliced
- Sea salt and black pepper to taste

Directions:

1. Heat olive oil in a large skillet over medium heat.
2. Add the garlic slices and sauté for 1-2 minutes until fragrant but not browned.
3. Add the spinach to the skillet, tossing gently with tongs to coat in the garlic oil.
4. Cook for 2-3 minutes, stirring occasionally, until the spinach is wilted.
5. Season with salt and pepper to taste, then serve immediately.

Nutritional value per serving: Calories: 120, Carbs: 3g, Fiber: 2g, Sugars: 1g, Protein: 2g, Saturated fat: 1g, Unsaturated fat: 10g

Difficulty rating: ★☆☆☆☆

Tips for ingredient variations: Add a squeeze of lemon juice before serving for a fresh, tangy twist.

Zucchini Fries (Oven-Baked)

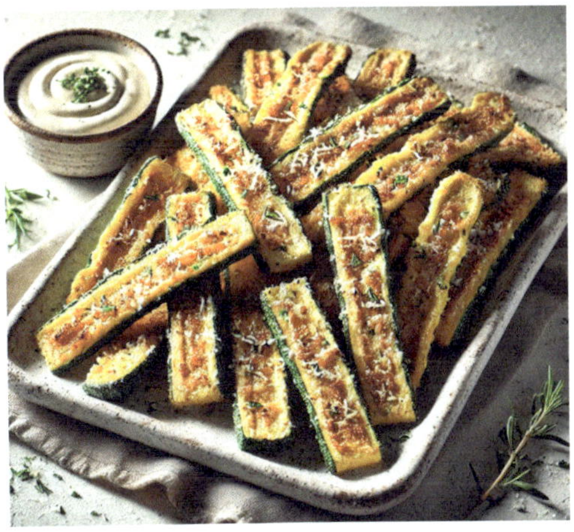

Number of servings: 4

Preparation time: 10 minutes

Cooking time: 20 minutes

Ingredients:

- 2 medium zucchinis, cut into fry-sized sticks
- 1/2 cup almond flour
- 1/4 cup grated Parmesan cheese
- 1 tsp smoked paprika
- 1/2 tsp garlic powder
- 2 large eggs, beaten
- Sea salt and black pepper to taste

Directions:

1. Preheat the oven to 425°F (220°C) and line a baking sheet with parchment paper.
2. In a shallow dish, mix almond flour, Parmesan, smoked paprika, garlic powder, salt, and pepper.
3. Coat each zucchini stick with the almond flour mixture after dipping it into the beaten eggs.
4. Place the coated zucchini sticks on the prepared baking sheet.
5. Bake for 20 minutes, flipping halfway through, until golden and crispy.
6. Serve warm with a low-carb dipping sauce.

Nutritional value per serving: Calories: 120, Carbs: 5g, Fiber: 2g, Sugars: 2g, Protein: 6g, Saturated fat: 2g, Unsaturated fat: 6g

Difficulty rating: ★★☆☆☆

Tips for ingredient variations: Add Italian seasoning or cayenne pepper to the coating for extra flavor.

Mashed Cauliflower with Butter

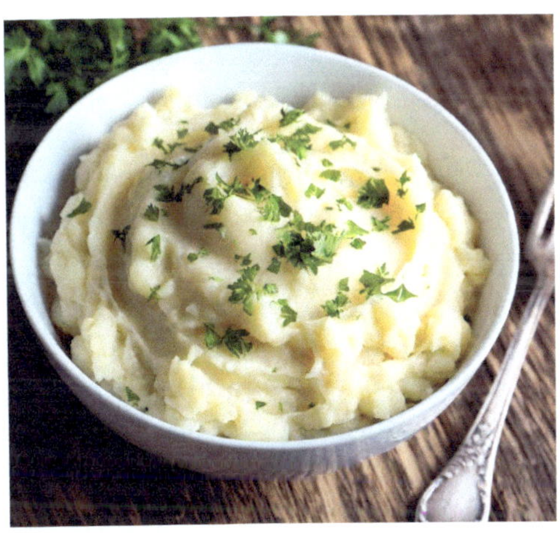

Number of servings: 4

Preparation time: 10 minutes

Cooking time: 15 minutes

Ingredients:

- 1 medium head of cauliflower, cut into florets
- 2 tbsp unsalted butter
- 1/4 cup heavy cream
- 1/4 cup grated Parmesan cheese (optional)
- Sea salt and black pepper to taste

Directions:

1. Bring a large pot of water to a boil and cook the cauliflower florets for 10-12 minutes, or until tender. Drain well.
2. Place the cooked cauliflower in a blender or food processor. Add butter, heavy cream, salt, and pepper.
3. Blend until smooth and creamy. Adjust seasoning to taste.
4. If desired, fold in Parmesan cheese for added flavor.
5. Serve warm as a low-carb alternative to mashed potatoes.

Nutritional value per serving: Calories: 110, Carbs: 5g, Fiber: 2g, Sugars: 2g, Protein: 4g, Saturated fat: 4g, Unsaturated fat: 2g

Difficulty rating: ★☆☆☆☆

Tips for ingredient variations: Mix in roasted garlic or fresh herbs like chives or parsley for extra depth of flavor.

Grilled Asparagus with Lemon Zest

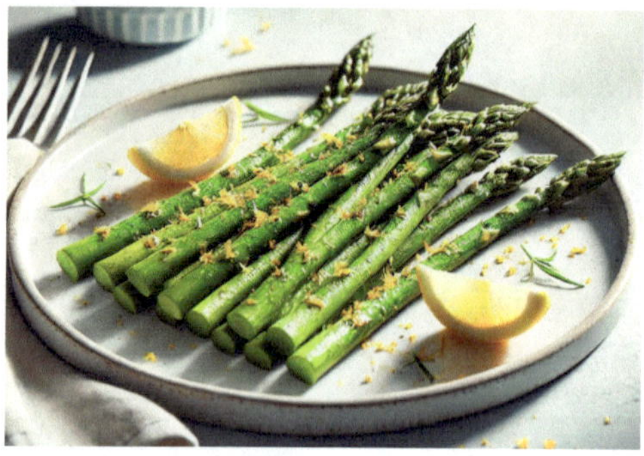

Number of servings: 4

Preparation time: 5 minutes

Cooking time: 10 minutes

Ingredients:

- 1 lb fresh asparagus, trimmed
- 2 tbsp olive oil
- 1 tsp lemon zest
- Sea salt and black pepper to taste

Directions:

1. Preheat a grill or grill pan over medium-high heat.
2. Add salt, pepper, and olive oil to the asparagus.
3. The asparagus should be soft and faintly browned after 5 to 7 minutes on the grill, rotating occasionally.
4. Transfer to a serving plate and sprinkle with lemon zest before serving.

Nutritional value per serving: Calories: 80, Carbs: 4g, Fiber: 2g, Sugars: 2g, Protein: 2g, Saturated fat: 1g, Unsaturated fat: 6g

Difficulty rating: ★☆☆☆☆

Tips for ingredient variations: Top with shaved Parmesan or toasted almonds for a more indulgent dish

Creamed Spinach (Low-Carb Version)

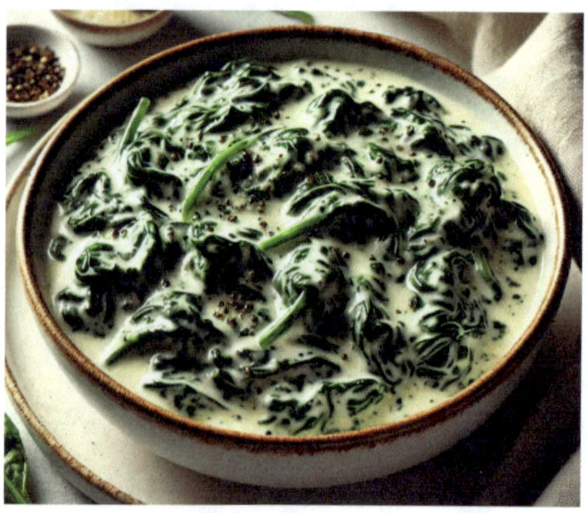

Number of servings: 4

Preparation time: 5 minutes

Cooking time: 10 minutes

Ingredients:

- 4 cups fresh spinach leaves
- 1/2 cup heavy cream
- 1/3 cup grated Parmesan cheese
- 2 tbsp cream cheese
- 1 tbsp butter
- 1 garlic clove, minced
- Sea salt and black pepper to taste

Directions:

1. Heat butter in a large skillet over medium heat. Add garlic and sauté for 1 minute until fragrant.
2. Add spinach and cook, stirring, until wilted (about 2-3 minutes).
3. Reduce the heat to low and stir in heavy cream, cream cheese, and Parmesan. Cook for another 2-3 minutes until the mixture thickens slightly.
4. Season with salt and pepper to taste. Serve warm.

Nutritional value per serving: Calories: 140, Carbs: 3g, Fiber: 1g, Sugars: 1g, Protein: 6g, Saturated fat: 8g, Unsaturated fat: 2g

Difficulty rating: ★☆☆☆☆

Tips for ingredient variations: Add sautéed mushrooms or crumbled bacon for additional flavor and texture.

Roasted Broccoli with Almonds

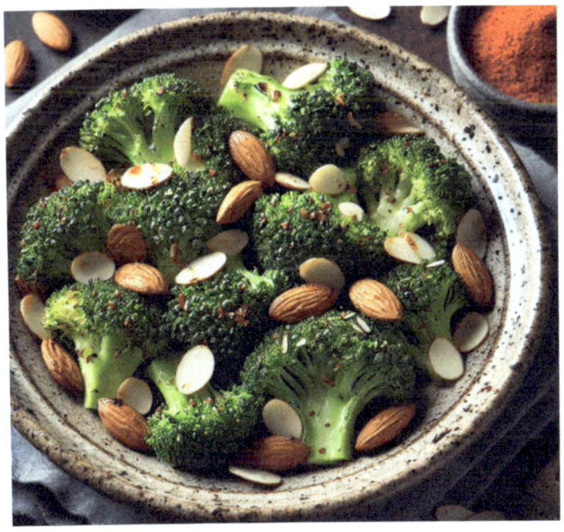

Number of servings: 4

Preparation time: 5 minutes

Cooking time: 20 minutes

Ingredients:

- 1 large head of broccoli, cut into florets
- 2 tbsp olive oil
- 1/4 cup sliced almonds
- 1/2 tsp garlic powder
- Sea salt and black pepper to taste

Directions:

1. Preheat the oven to 400°F (200°C).
2. Broccoli florets should be tossed in a large mixing dish with olive oil, garlic powder, salt, and pepper.
3. Spread the broccoli evenly on a baking sheet. Roast for 15 minutes, stirring halfway through.
4. Sprinkle almonds over the broccoli and roast for an additional 5 minutes until the almonds are golden and broccoli is tender.
5. Serve immediately.

Nutritional value per serving: Calories: 120, Carbs: 6g, Fiber: 3g, Sugars: 2g, Protein: 4g, Saturated fat: 1g, Unsaturated fat: 7g

Difficulty rating: ★☆☆☆☆

Tips for ingredient variations: Add a sprinkle of grated Parmesan or a squeeze of lemon juice for extra flavor.

Cauliflower Rice Pilaf

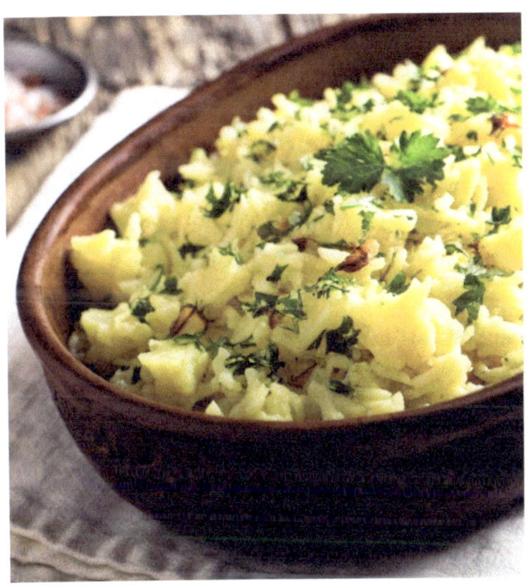

Number of servings: 4

Preparation time: 10 minutes

Cooking time: 10 minutes

Ingredients:

- 4 cups cauliflower rice (store-bought or homemade)
- 2 tbsp olive oil
- 1 small onion, finely diced
- 1 garlic clove, minced
- 1/4 cup sliced almonds
- 2 tbsp fresh parsley, chopped
- 1 tsp ground cumin
- Sea salt and black pepper to taste

Directions:

1. Heat olive oil in a large skillet over medium heat. Add onion and garlic, sautéing until softened (about 3 minutes).
2. Add cauliflower rice and cumin. Cook for 5-7 minutes, stirring occasionally, until tender.
3. Stir in almonds and parsley. Season with salt and pepper to taste.
4. Serve as a side dish or base for a protein-rich meal.

Nutritional value per serving: Calories: 90, Carbs: 6g, Fiber: 2g, Sugars: 2g, Protein: 3g, Saturated fat: 1g, Unsaturated fat: 5g

Difficulty rating: ★☆☆☆☆

Tips for ingredient variations: Incorporate dried cranberries or pine nuts for a slightly different flavor profile.

Baked Spaghetti Squash with Parmesan

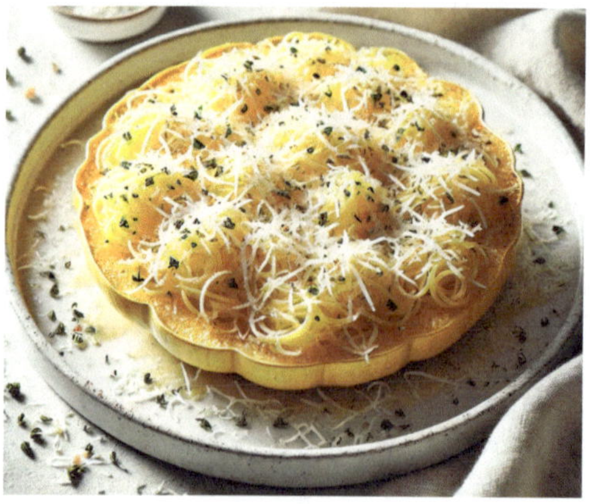

Number of servings: 4

Preparation time: 10 minutes

Cooking time: 40 minutes

Ingredients:

- 1 medium spaghetti squash
- 2 tbsp olive oil
- 1/2 cup grated Parmesan cheese
- 1 tsp garlic powder
- 1/2 tsp dried oregano
- Sea salt and black pepper to taste

Directions:

1. Preheat the oven to 400°F (200°C).
2. After halving the spaghetti squash lengthwise, remove the seeds with a spoon. Drizzle olive oil over the cut sides and sprinkle with garlic powder, oregano, salt, and pepper.
3. Place the squash halves cut-side down on a baking sheet and roast for 30-35 minutes, or until tender.
4. Use a fork to scrape the squash into spaghetti-like strands. Sprinkle with Parmesan cheese and mix gently. Serve warm.

Nutritional value per serving: Calories: 120, Carbs: 8g, Fiber: 2g, Sugars: 4g, Protein: 6g, Saturated fat: 2g, Unsaturated fat: 6g

Difficulty rating: ★☆☆☆☆

Tips for ingredient variations: Top with marinara sauce or grilled chicken for a more filling meal.

Garlic Butter Mushrooms

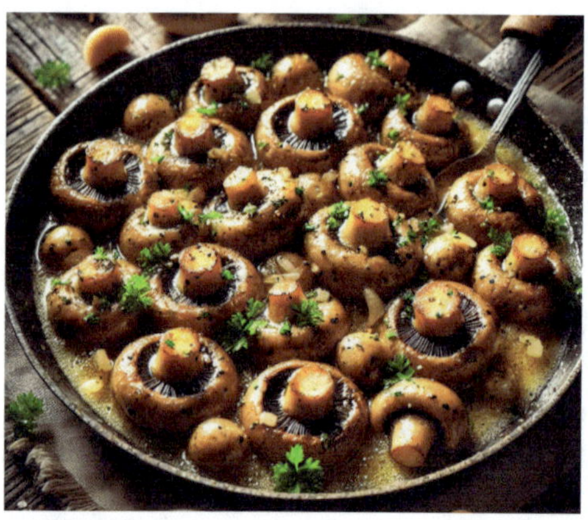

Number of servings: 4

Preparation time: 5 minutes

Cooking time: 10 minutes

Ingredients:

- 1 lb (450g) button mushrooms, cleaned and trimmed
- 3 tbsp butter
- 2 garlic cloves, minced
- 1 tbsp fresh parsley, chopped
- Sea salt and black pepper to taste

Directions:

1. Heat butter in a large skillet over medium heat. Add garlic and sauté for 1 minute until fragrant.
2. Add the mushrooms and cook until they are soft and golden brown, stirring periodically, for 8 to 10 minutes.
3. Season with salt and pepper to taste. Sprinkle with fresh parsley before serving.

Nutritional value per serving: Calories: 100, Carbs: 4g, Fiber: 1g, Sugars: 2g, Protein: 3g, Saturated fat: 6g, Unsaturated fat: 1g

Difficulty rating: ★☆☆☆☆

Tips for ingredient variations: Add a splash of white wine or a pinch of red pepper flakes for a more complex flavor.

Cucumber and Dill Salad

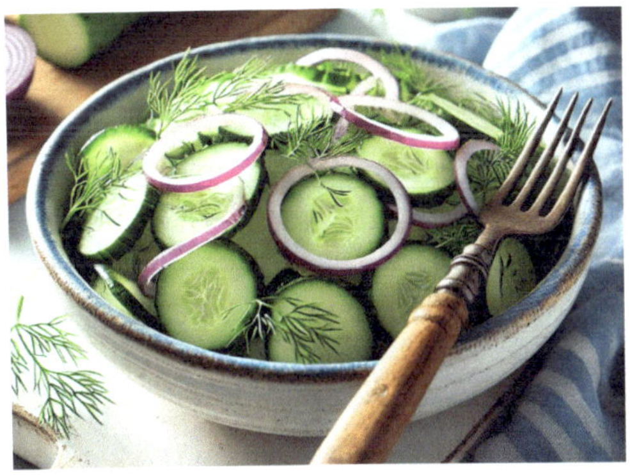

Number of servings: 2
Preparation time: 10 minutes
Cooking time: 0 minutes

Ingredients:

- 1 large cucumber, thinly sliced
- 2 tbsp fresh dill, chopped
- 2 tbsp Greek yogurt (unsweetened)
- 1 tbsp lemon juice
- 1 tsp olive oil
- Sea salt and black pepper to taste

Directions:

1. In a large bowl, combine the cucumber slices and chopped dill.
2. In a separate small bowl, whisk together the Greek yogurt, lemon juice, olive oil, salt, and pepper to make the dressing.
3. Pour the dressing over the cucumber and dill mixture. Toss gently to coat evenly.
4. Serve immediately or chill for 15 minutes for a refreshing option.

Nutritional value per serving: Calories: 60, Carbs: 4g, Fiber: 1g, Sugars: 2g, Protein: 3g, Saturated fat: 1g, Unsaturated fat: 1g

Difficulty rating: ★☆☆☆☆

Tips for ingredient variations: Add thinly sliced red onion or crumbled feta for an extra flavor boost.

Sautéed Green Beans with Bacon Bits

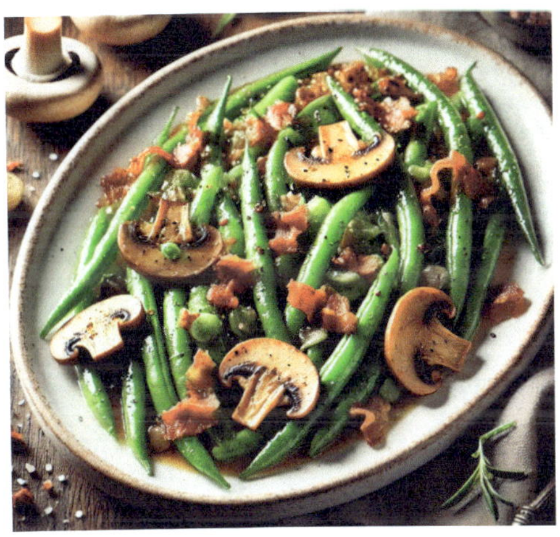

Number of servings: 2
Preparation time: 5 minutes
Cooking time: 10 minutes

Ingredients:

- 200g fresh green beans, trimmed
- 2 slices of bacon, cooked and crumbled
- 1 tbsp olive oil or butter
- 1 garlic clove, minced
- Sea salt and black pepper to taste

Directions:

1. Heat the olive oil or butter in a skillet over medium heat.
2. Add the green beans and sauté for 5-7 minutes, stirring occasionally, until tender but still crisp.
3. Add the minced garlic and cook for an additional 1-2 minutes until fragrant.
4. Remove from heat and sprinkle with the crumbled bacon. Season with salt and pepper, then toss gently to combine.
5. Serve warm.

Nutritional value per serving: Calories: 120, Carbs: 5g, Fiber: 2g, Sugars: 2g, Protein: 6g, Saturated fat: 3g, Unsaturated fat: 4g

Difficulty rating: ★☆☆☆☆

Tips for ingredient variations: Add a splash of lemon juice or a sprinkle of parmesan cheese for added flavor.

Crispy Kale Chips

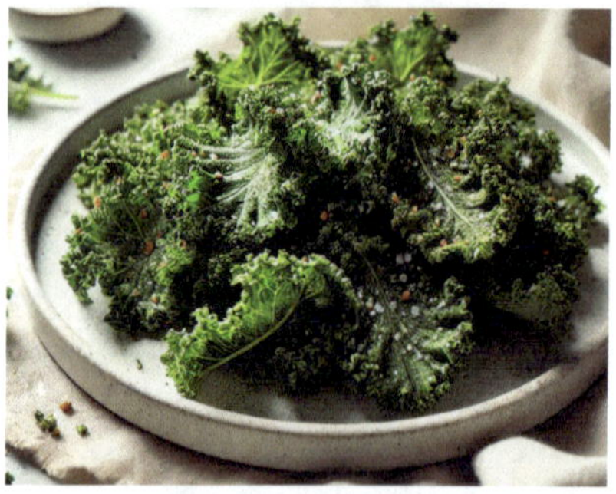

Number of servings: 2
Preparation time: 5 minutes
Cooking time: 15 minutes

Ingredients:

- 150g kale, washed and dried, stems removed
- 1 tbsp olive oil
- 1/2 tsp sea salt
- 1/2 tsp smoked paprika or garlic powder (optional)

Directions:

1. Preheat the oven to 325°F (160°C) and line a baking sheet with parchment paper.
2. Tear the kale into bite-sized pieces and place in a large bowl.
3. Drizzle the kale with olive oil, then rub it into the leaves until they are equally covered.
4. Spread the kale on the baking sheet in a single layer. Sprinkle with salt and optional seasonings.
5. Bake for 12-15 minutes, checking frequently to prevent burning, until the kale is crisp.
6. Let cool slightly before serving.

Nutritional value per serving: Calories: 70, Carbs: 4g, Fiber: 2g, Sugars: 1g, Protein: 3g, Saturated fat: 0g, Unsaturated fat: 3g

Difficulty rating: ★☆☆☆☆

Tips for ingredient variations: Add nutritional yeast for a cheesy flavor or chili flakes for a spicy kick.

Roasted Radishes with Herbs

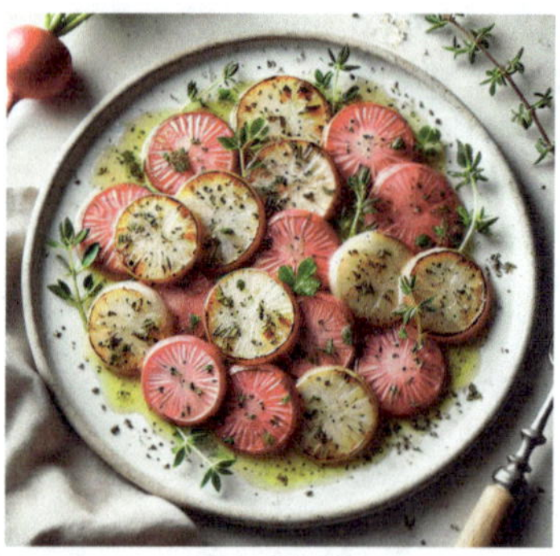

Number of servings: 2
Preparation time: 5 minutes
Cooking time: 20 minutes

Ingredients:

- 1 bunch of radishes, trimmed and halved
- 1 tbsp olive oil
- 1 tsp fresh thyme or rosemary, chopped
- Sea salt and black pepper to taste

Directions:

1. Preheat the oven to 400°F (200°C) and line a baking sheet with parchment paper.
2. In a bowl, toss the radish halves with olive oil, thyme, salt, and pepper.
3. Spread the radishes in a single layer on the baking sheet.
4. Roast for 18-20 minutes, stirring halfway through, until tender and lightly browned.
5. Serve warm as a side dish or snack.

Nutritional value per serving: Calories: 45, Carbs: 4g, Fiber: 2g, Sugars: 2g, Protein: 1g, Saturated fat: 0g, Unsaturated fat: 3g

Difficulty rating: ★☆☆☆☆

Tips for ingredient variations: Drizzle with a balsamic glaze for a touch of sweetness or sprinkle with parmesan cheese before serving.

Caprese Salad Skewers

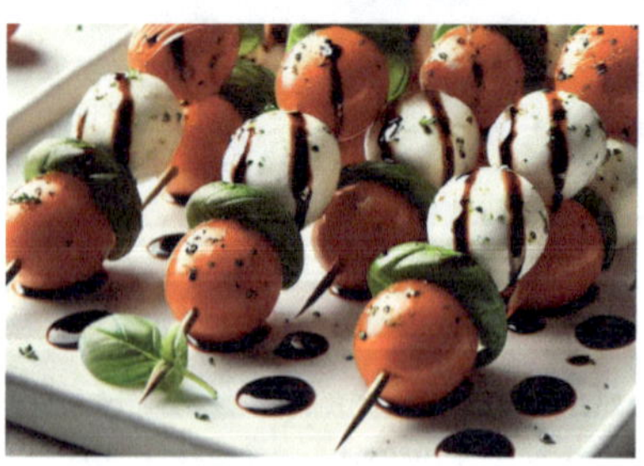

Number of servings: 4
Preparation time: 10 minutes
Cooking time: 0 minutes

Ingredients:

- 16 cherry tomatoes
- 16 small mozzarella balls (bocconcini)
- 16 fresh basil leaves
- 2 tbsp balsamic glaze
- 1 tbsp olive oil
- Sea salt and black pepper to taste
- 16 small skewers or toothpicks

Directions:

1. Thread one mozzarella ball, one cherry tomato, and one basil leaf onto each skewer to assemble the skewers.
2. Arrange the skewers on a serving platter.
3. Drizzle with balsamic glaze and olive oil. Sprinkle with salt and pepper to taste.
4. Serve immediately as an appetizer or snack.

Nutritional value per serving (4 skewers): Calories: 120, Carbs: 3g, Fiber: 0g, Sugars: 2g, Protein: 6g, Saturated fat: 3g, Unsaturated fat: 4g

Difficulty rating: ★☆☆☆☆

Tips for ingredient variations: Add a slice of prosciutto for an extra protein boost or use marinated mozzarella for enhanced flavor.

Snacks

Deviled Eggs with Avocado

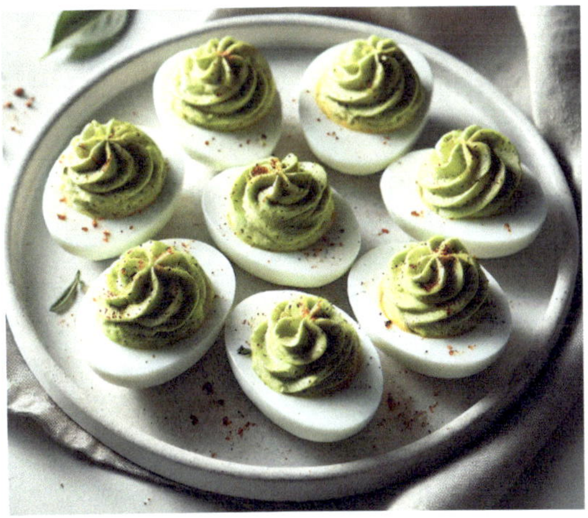

Number of servings: 4

Preparation time: 15 minutes

Cooking time: 10 minutes

Ingredients:

- 4 large eggs
- 1 ripe avocado, mashed
- 1 tsp lime juice
- 1 tbsp mayonnaise (optional)
- 1/2 tsp garlic powder
- Sea salt and black pepper to taste
- Paprika for garnish

Directions:

1. Place the eggs in a saucepan, cover with water, and bring to a boil. Once boiling, reduce heat and simmer for 10 minutes.
2. Transfer the eggs to an ice bath and let cool. Peel the shells once cooled.
3. Slice the eggs in half lengthwise and remove the yolks, placing them in a bowl.
4. Mash the yolks with the avocado, lime juice, mayonnaise (if using), garlic powder, salt, and pepper until smooth.
5. Spoon the mixture back into the egg whites.
6. Sprinkle with paprika and serve immediately or refrigerate until ready to serve.

Nutritional value per serving: Calories: 120, Carbs: 2g, Fiber: 1g, Sugars: 0g, Protein: 6g, Saturated fat: 2g, Unsaturated fat: 5g

Difficulty rating: ★☆☆☆☆

Tips for ingredient variations: Add a touch of hot sauce for spice or finely chopped fresh herbs like parsley or chives for extra flavor.

Celery Sticks with Peanut Butter

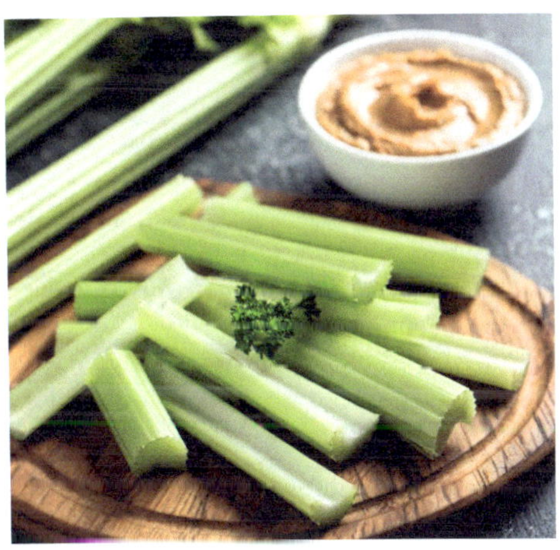

Number of servings: 2

Preparation time: 5 minutes

Cooking time: 0 minutes

Ingredients:

- 4 celery sticks
- 2 tbsp natural peanut butter (no added sugar or oils)
- 1 tbsp chia seeds or crushed nuts for topping (optional)

Directions:

1. Wash and trim the celery sticks.
2. Spread 1/2 tbsp of peanut butter into each celery stick.
3. Sprinkle with chia seeds or crushed nuts for added texture and nutrition.
4. Serve immediately.

Nutritional value per serving: Calories: 150, Carbs: 5g, Fiber: 3g, Sugars: 2g, Protein: 6g, Saturated fat: 1g, Unsaturated fat: 4g

Difficulty rating: ★☆☆☆☆

Tips for ingredient variations: Swap peanut butter with almond butter or sunflower seed butter for different flavor profiles.

Cheese Crisps (Oven-Baked)

Number of servings: 4
Preparation time: 5 minutes
Cooking time: 8-10 minutes

Ingredients:

- 1 cup shredded cheese (cheddar, Parmesan, or a mix)
- 1/2 tsp paprika or garlic powder (optional)

Directions:

1. Preheat your oven to 375°F (190°C) and line a baking sheet with parchment paper.
2. Arrange heaps of shredded cheese on the baking sheet, about 2 inches apart, in tablespoon-sized mounds.
3. Sprinkle with paprika or garlic powder for added flavor, if desired.
4. Bake for 8-10 minutes, or until the cheese crisps are golden and bubbly.
5. Allow to cool on the baking sheet for 5 minutes before transferring to a plate.

Nutritional value per serving: Calories: 100, Carbs: 1g, Fiber: 0g, Sugars: 0g, Protein: 8g, Saturated fat: 5g, Unsaturated fat: 2g

Difficulty rating: ★☆☆☆☆

Tips for ingredient variations: Use different cheeses like Gruyère or Asiago for unique flavor profiles.

Almonds, Pecans, and Pumpkin Seed Mix with Coconut Flakes

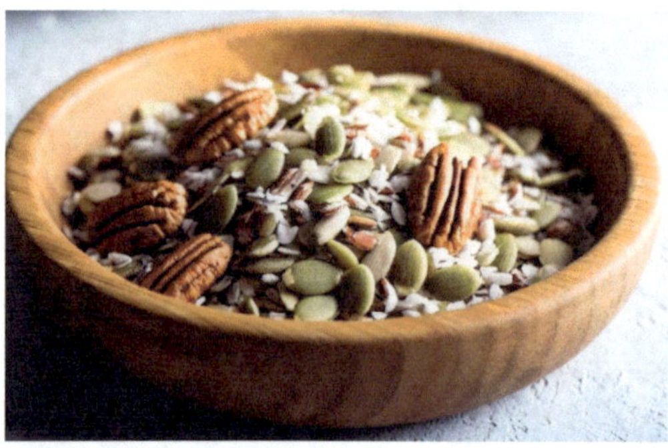

Number of servings: 4
Preparation time: 5 minutes
Cooking time: 0 minutes

Ingredients:

- 1/2 cup raw almonds
- 1/2 cup raw pecans
- 1/4 cup raw pumpkin seeds
- 1/4 cup unsweetened coconut flakes
- 1/2 tsp cinnamon or cocoa powder (optional)

Directions:

1. Combine almonds, pecans, pumpkin seeds, and coconut flakes in a bowl.
2. Add cinnamon or cocoa powder, if using, and toss until evenly coated.
3. Store in an airtight container and serve as a snack.

Nutritional value per serving: Calories: 200, Carbs: 4g, Fiber: 2g, Sugars: 1g, Protein: 5g, Saturated fat: 4g, Unsaturated fat: 12g

Difficulty rating: ★☆☆☆☆

Tips for ingredient variations: Add a handful of freeze-dried berries for a tart, low-sugar contrast.

Turkey Jerky

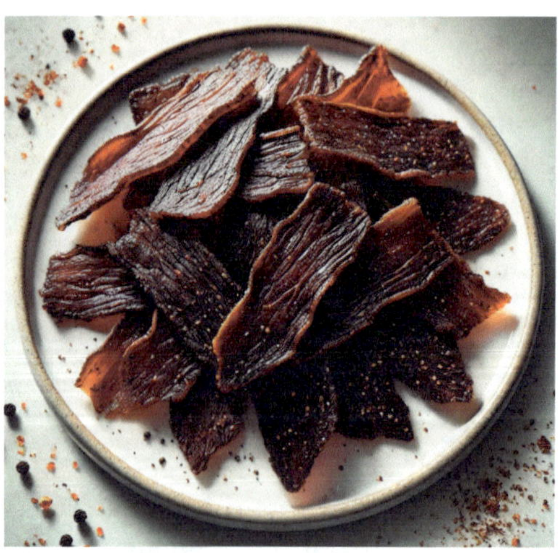

Number of servings: 6
Preparation time: 15 minutes
Cooking time: 4-5 hours (dehydrator or oven)

Ingredients:

- 1 lb turkey breast, thinly sliced
- 1/4 cup soy sauce or coconut aminos
- 1 tbsp apple cider vinegar
- 1 tsp garlic powder
- 1 tsp smoked paprika
- 1/2 tsp black pepper

Directions:

1. In a bowl, mix soy sauce (or coconut aminos), apple cider vinegar, garlic powder, smoked paprika, and black pepper.
2. Add the turkey slices to the marinade, ensuring all pieces are coated. Marinate for at least 2 hours, preferably overnight.
3. Preheat your oven to 170°F (or use a food dehydrator).
4. On a wire rack set over a baking sheet, arrange the turkey slices in a single layer.
5. Dry in the oven or dehydrator for 4-5 hours, flipping halfway through, until the turkey is fully dried and chewy.
6. Store in an airtight container for up to a week.

Nutritional value per serving: Calories: 70, Carbs: 1g, Fiber: 0g, Sugars: 0g, Protein: 12g, Saturated fat: 0g, Unsaturated fat: 1g

Difficulty rating: ★★★☆☆

Tips for ingredient variations: Add red pepper flakes or a dash of honey for a spicy-sweet twist.

Guacamole with Bell Pepper Slices

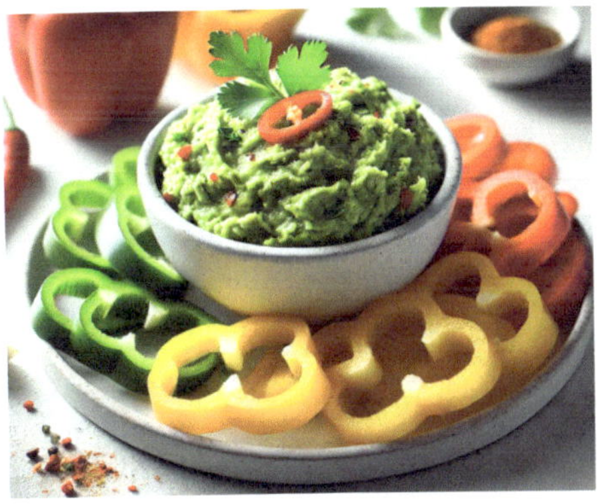

Number of servings: 2
Preparation time: 10 minutes
Cooking time: 0 minutes

Ingredients:

- 1 ripe avocado
- 1 tbsp lime juice
- 1 small garlic clove, minced
- 1 tbsp fresh cilantro, chopped
- 1/2 tsp sea salt
- 1/4 tsp chili powder (optional)
- 2 medium bell peppers (any color), sliced

Directions:

1. Scoop the avocado's flesh into a bowl after halves it and removing the pit.
2. Add lime juice, minced garlic, chopped cilantro, salt, and chili powder if desired. Mash with a fork until creamy but slightly chunky.
3. Arrange the bell pepper slices on a plate and serve alongside the guacamole.

Nutritional value per serving: Calories: 120, Carbs: 8g, Fiber: 5g, Sugars: 3g, Protein: 2g, Saturated fat: 1g, Unsaturated fat: 10g

Difficulty rating: ★☆☆☆☆

Tips for ingredient variations: Add diced tomatoes or red onions to the guacamole for extra texture and flavor.

Hard-Boiled Eggs with Mustard

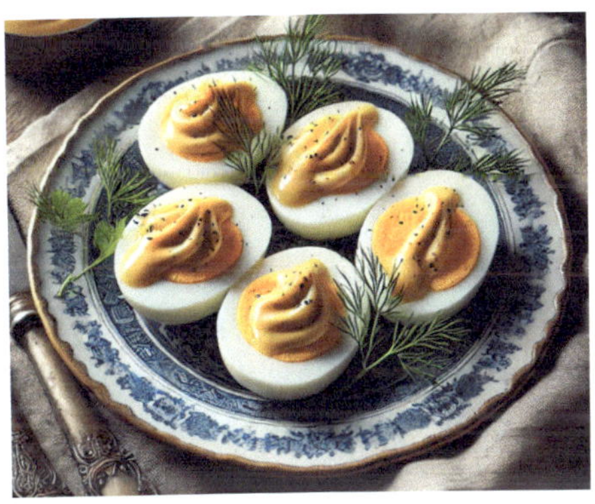

Number of servings: 2
Preparation time: 5 minutes
Cooking time: 10 minutes

Ingredients:

- 4 large eggs
- 1 tbsp Dijon mustard
- 1 tsp olive oil
- Sea salt and black pepper to taste

Directions:

1. Place the eggs in a saucepan and cover with water. Bring to a boil, then reduce the heat to low and simmer for 9-10 minutes.
2. Drain the hot water and transfer the eggs to an ice bath to cool for 5 minutes. Peel the eggs.
3. Slice the eggs in half and drizzle with olive oil and a dollop of Dijon mustard. Season with salt and pepper to taste.

Nutritional value per serving: Calories: 140, Carbs: 1g, Fiber: 0g, Sugars: 0g, Protein: 12g, Saturated fat: 3g, Unsaturated fat: 7g

Difficulty rating: ★☆☆☆☆

Tips for ingredient variations: Sprinkle with smoked paprika or fresh herbs like chives for added flavor.

Cottage Cheese with Paprika

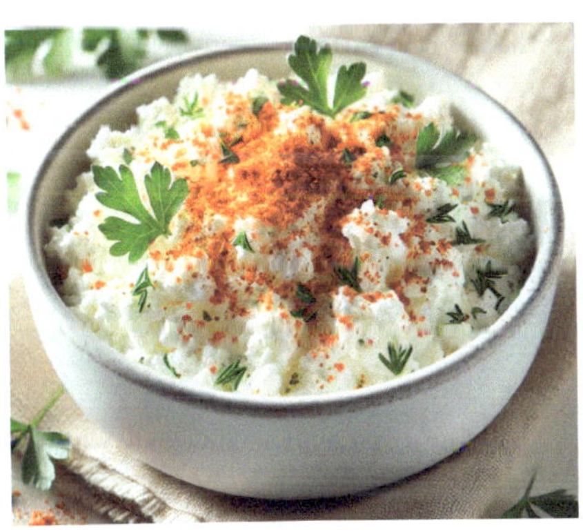

Number of servings: 1
Preparation time: 5 minutes
Cooking time: 0 minutes

Ingredients:

- 1 cup low-fat cottage cheese
- 1/2 tsp smoked paprika
- 1/4 tsp garlic powder (optional)
- 1 tbsp fresh parsley, chopped

Directions:

1. Spoon the cottage cheese into a serving bowl.
2. Sprinkle with smoked paprika, garlic powder if desired, and fresh parsley.
3. Serve immediately or refrigerate until ready to eat.

Nutritional value per serving: Calories: 120, Carbs: 4g, Fiber: 0g, Sugars: 2g, Protein: 20g, Saturated fat: 2g, Unsaturated fat: 1g

Difficulty rating: ★☆☆☆☆

Tips for ingredient variations: Top with a handful of sliced cherry tomatoes or cucumber for extra freshness.

Spicy Roasted Chickpeas with Turmeric

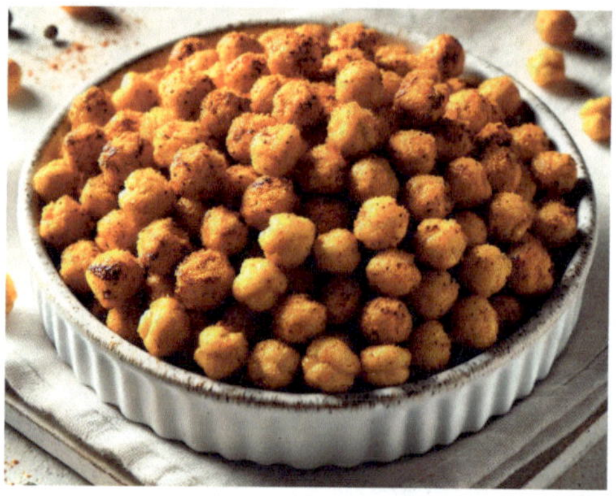

Number of servings: 4

Preparation time: 10 minutes

Cooking time: 25 minutes

Ingredients:

- 1 can (15 oz) chickpeas, drained and rinsed
- 1 tbsp extra virgin olive oil
- 1 tsp ground turmeric
- 1/2 tsp smoked paprika
- 1/2 tsp ground cumin
- 1/4 tsp cayenne pepper (optional, for added heat)
- 1/2 tsp garlic powder
- Sea salt and black pepper to taste

Directions:

1. Preheat the oven to 400°F (200°C) and line a baking sheet with parchment paper.
2. Pat the chickpeas dry with a clean kitchen towel or paper towels. Removing excess moisture ensures they crisp up nicely during roasting.
3. In a large mixing bowl, toss the chickpeas with olive oil, turmeric, smoked paprika, cumin, cayenne (if using), garlic powder, salt, and pepper until evenly coated.
4. Spread the seasoned chickpeas in a single layer on the prepared baking sheet.
5. Roast in the preheated oven for 20–25 minutes, stirring halfway through, until the chickpeas are golden and crispy.
6. Allow to cool slightly before serving. Store leftovers in an airtight container at room temperature for up to 3 days.

Nutritional value per serving: Calories: 110, Carbs: 15g, Fiber: 4g, Sugars: 1g, Protein: 5g, Saturated fat: 0.5g, Unsaturated fat: 2.5g

Difficulty rating: ★☆☆☆☆

Tips for ingredient variations: For a slightly sweet twist, add a pinch of cinnamon to the spice blend. To enhance crunch, sprinkle the roasted chickpeas with sesame seeds after baking.

Olives and Cheese Cubes

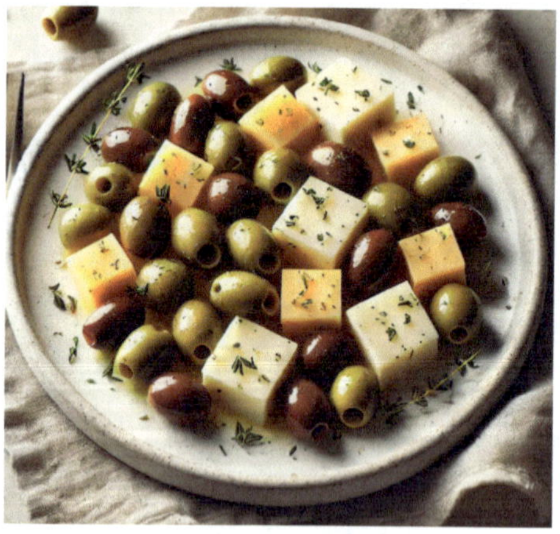

Number of servings: 2

Preparation time: 5 minutes

Cooking time: 0 minutes

Ingredients:

- 1/2 cup mixed olives (black and green)
- 1/2 cup cheese cubes (cheddar, Gouda, or Monterey Jack)
- 1 tsp olive oil
- 1/4 tsp dried oregano

Directions:

1. Toss the olives and cheese cubes in a bowl with olive oil and dried oregano.
2. Serve immediately as a quick snack or appetizer.

Nutritional value per serving: Calories: 190, Carbs: 2g, Fiber: 1g, Sugars: 0g, Protein: 8g, Saturated fat: 5g, Unsaturated fat: 7g

Difficulty rating: ★☆☆☆☆

Tips for ingredient variations: Add a handful of cherry tomatoes or cucumber slices for extra texture and flavor.

Keto Fat Bombs (Coconut Oil and Cocoa)

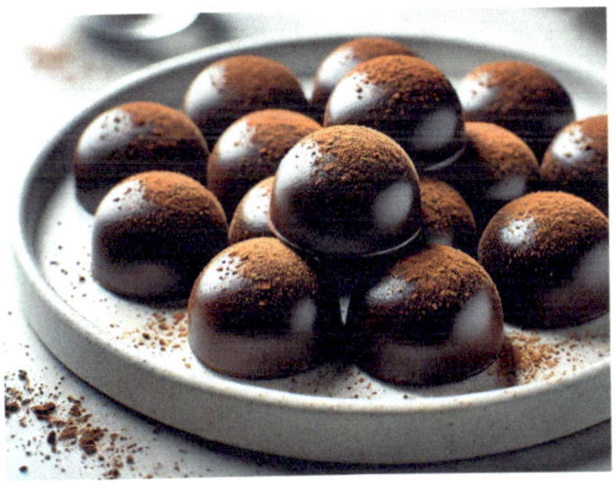

Number of servings: 10
Preparation time: 10 minutes
Cooking time: 0 minutes (chill for 1 hour)

Ingredients:

- 1/2 cup coconut oil, melted
- 1/4 cup unsweetened cocoa powder
- 2 tbsp almond butter or peanut butter (sugar-free)
- 1 tbsp erythritol or monk fruit sweetener
- 1/2 tsp vanilla extract
- Pinch of sea salt

Directions:

1. In a mixing bowl, combine the melted coconut oil, cocoa powder, almond butter, sweetener, vanilla extract, and sea salt. Whisk until smooth.
2. Pour the mixture into silicone molds or mini cupcake liners.
3. Place the molds in the freezer for 1 hour or until the fat bombs are firm.
4. Pop out the fat bombs and store them in an airtight container in the freezer. Enjoy chilled.

Nutritional value per serving: Calories: 90, Carbs: 2g, Fiber: 1g, Sugars: 0g, Protein: 1g, Saturated fat: 8g, Unsaturated fat: 1g

Difficulty rating: ★☆☆☆☆

Tips for ingredient variations: Add a sprinkle of unsweetened shredded coconut or chopped nuts for texture.

Sliced Cucumber with Cream Cheese

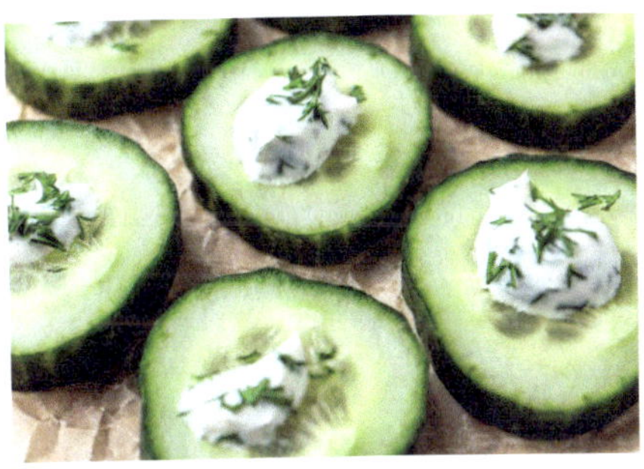

Number of servings: 2
Preparation time: 5 minutes
Cooking time: 0 minutes

Ingredients:

- 1 large cucumber, sliced into rounds
- 4 tbsp cream cheese, softened
- 1 tbsp fresh dill, chopped
- 1 tsp garlic powder
- Pinch of sea salt and black pepper

Directions:

1. Spread a thin layer of cream cheese on each cucumber slice.
2. Sprinkle with fresh dill, garlic powder, salt, and pepper.
3. Arrange on a platter and serve immediately.

Nutritional value per serving: Calories: 80, Carbs: 3g, Fiber: 1g, Sugars: 1g, Protein: 2g, Saturated fat: 4g, Unsaturated fat: 2g

Difficulty rating: ★☆☆☆☆

Tips for ingredient variations: Top with smoked salmon or a small slice of turkey for extra protein.

Zucchini Chips (Baked with Olive Oil)

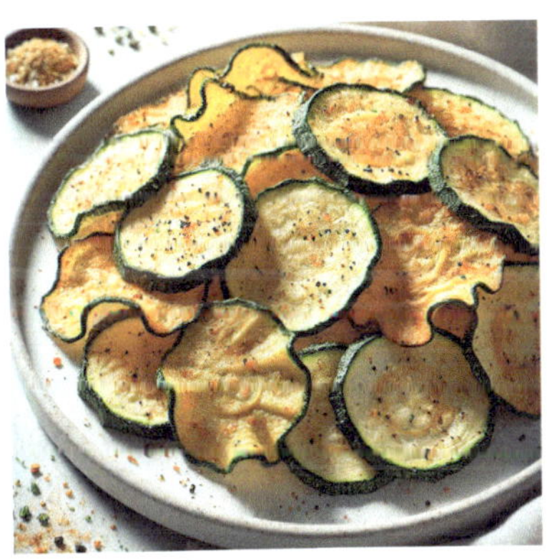

Number of servings: 2
Preparation time: 10 minutes
Cooking time: 30 minutes

Ingredients:

- 2 medium zucchinis, thinly sliced
- 1 tbsp olive oil
- 1/2 tsp garlic powder
- 1/2 tsp smoked paprika
- Sea salt to taste

Directions:

1. Preheat your oven to 200°F (90°C) and line a baking sheet with parchment paper.
2. Toss the zucchini slices with olive oil, garlic powder, smoked paprika, and salt in a bowl.
3. Arrange the slices in a single layer on the baking sheet.
4. Bake for 30 minutes or until crispy, flipping halfway through.
5. Allow to cool slightly before serving.

Nutritional value per serving: Calories: 70, Carbs: 5g, Fiber: 1g, Sugars: 2g, Protein: 1g, Saturated fat: 1g, Unsaturated fat: 6g

Difficulty rating: ★★☆☆☆

Tips for ingredient variations: Add grated Parmesan before baking for a cheesy twist.

Low-Carb Trail Mix (Nuts and Seeds)

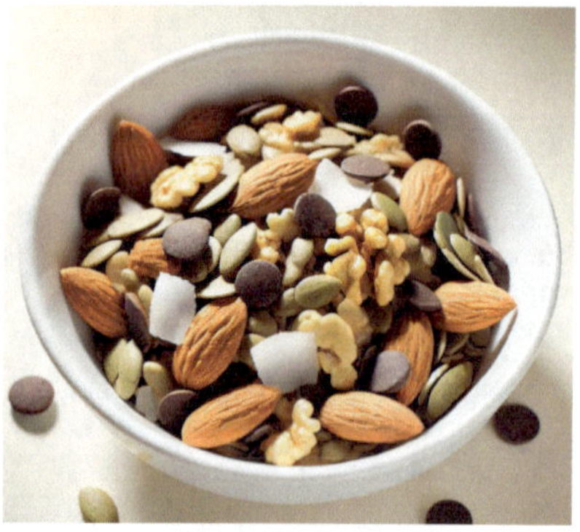

Number of servings: 4

Preparation time: 5 minutes

Cooking time: 0 minutes

Ingredients:

- 1/4 cup almonds
- 1/4 cup walnuts
- 1/4 cup pumpkin seeds
- 1/4 cup sunflower seeds
- 2 tbsp unsweetened coconut flakes
- 2 tbsp dark chocolate chips (sugar-free)

Directions:

1. Combine all the ingredients in a mixing bowl.
2. Portion into small snack bags or store in an airtight container for easy access.

Nutritional value per serving: Calories: 180, Carbs: 5g, Fiber: 3g, Sugars: 1g, Protein: 6g, Saturated fat: 3g, Unsaturated fat: 10g

Difficulty rating: ★☆☆☆☆

Tips for ingredient variations: Add a pinch of cinnamon or cayenne for extra flavor.

Mini Meatballs with Tomato Dipping Sauce

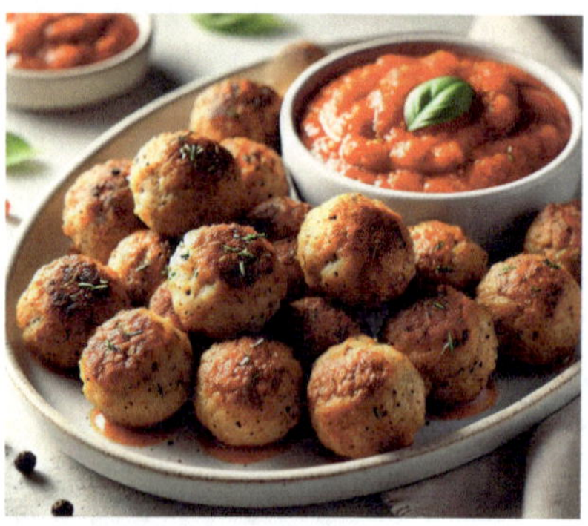

Number of servings: 4

Preparation time: 15 minutes

Cooking time: 15 minutes

Ingredients:

- 1 lb ground turkey or lean ground beef
- 1 large egg
- 2 tbsp almond flour
- 2 cloves garlic, minced
- 1 tsp dried oregano
- 1/2 tsp onion powder
- 1/2 tsp salt
- 1/4 tsp freshly ground black pepper
- 1 tbsp olive oil (for cooking)

For the Tomato Dipping Sauce:

- 1 cup crushed tomatoes (no sugar added)
- 1 tsp olive oil
- 1 clove garlic, minced
- 1/2 tsp dried basil
- 1/4 tsp chili flakes (optional)
- Salt and pepper to taste

Directions:

1. In a large mixing bowl, combine the ground turkey (or beef), egg, almond flour, minced garlic, oregano, onion powder, salt, and pepper. Mix gently until all ingredients are just combined.
2. Form the mixture into small meatballs, roughly 1 inch in diameter. You should have about 16 mini meatballs.
3. Heat olive oil in a large skillet over medium heat. To prevent crowding, add the meatballs and cook them in batches if needed. Sear them on all sides for about 6–8 minutes, turning occasionally, until browned and cooked through.
4. While the meatballs are cooking, prepare the tomato dipping sauce. In a small saucepan over medium heat, warm the olive oil and add the minced garlic. Sauté for 30 seconds until fragrant.
5. Stir in the crushed tomatoes, dried basil, chili flakes (if using), and a pinch of salt and pepper. Simmer until the sauce gradually thickens, 5 to 7 minutes, stirring periodically.
6. Transfer the meatballs to a serving plate and serve with the warm tomato dipping sauce on the side.

Nutritional value per serving: Calories: 210, Carbs: 6g, Fiber: 2g, Sugars: 3g, Protein: 22g, Saturated fat: 2g, Unsaturated fat: 5g

Difficulty rating: ★★☆☆☆

Tips for ingredient variations: For added flavor, mix fresh parsley or grated Parmesan cheese into the meatball mixture. If you prefer a dairy-free sauce, replace olive oil with avocado oil. For a spicier version, add extra chili flakes to the dipping sauce.

Desserts

Dark Chocolate Mousse with Whipped Cream

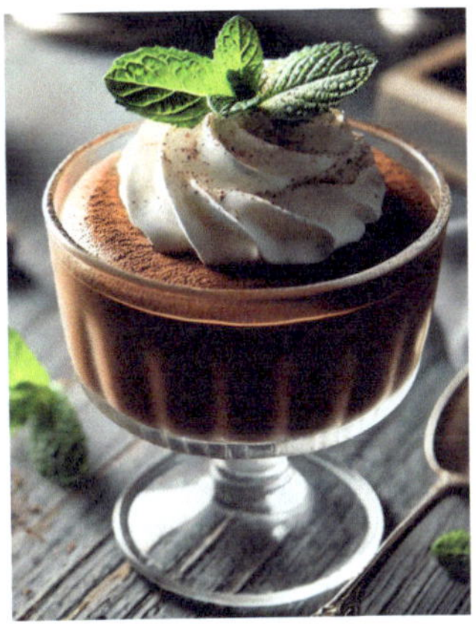

Number of servings: 4

Preparation time: 10 minutes

Cooking time: 0 minutes

Ingredients:

- 1 cup heavy cream (divided)
- 1/2 cup dark chocolate (85% cocoa or higher), chopped
- 1 tsp vanilla extract
- 2 tbsp powdered erythritol or stevia (adjust to taste)

Directions:

1. Heat 1/2 cup of heavy cream in a saucepan over low heat until warm, but not boiling.
2. Add the chopped dark chocolate to the warm cream and stir until fully melted and smooth. Allow to cool slightly.
3. In a mixing bowl, whisk the remaining heavy cream with the vanilla extract and powdered erythritol until soft peaks form.
4. Mix the whipped cream with the chilled chocolate mixture by gently folding them together.
5. Divide the mousse into serving cups and chill for at least 1 hour before serving.
6. Optionally, top with additional whipped cream before serving.

Nutritional value per serving: Calories: 210, Carbs: 6g, Fiber: 3g, Sugars: 1g, Protein: 3g, Saturated fat: 9g, Unsaturated fat: 2g

Difficulty rating: ★☆☆☆☆

Tips for ingredient variations: Add a pinch of sea salt or a dash of cinnamon for extra flavor.

Almond Flour Brownies

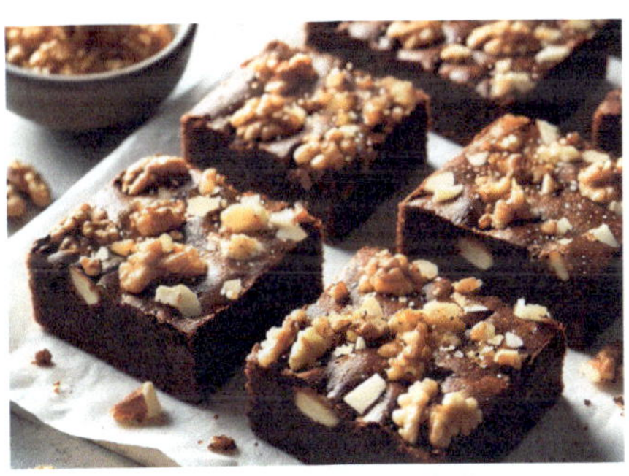

Number of servings: 12

Preparation time: 15 minutes

Cooking time: 20 minutes

Ingredients:

- 1 cup almond flour
- 1/2 cup unsweetened cocoa powder
- 1/2 tsp baking powder
- 1/4 tsp sea salt
- 1/2 cup unsalted butter, melted
- 1/2 cup erythritol or monk fruit sweetener
- 2 large eggs
- 1 tsp vanilla extract
- 1/4 cup dark chocolate chips (optional)

Directions:

1. Preheat the oven to 350°F (175°C) and line an 8x8-inch baking pan with parchment paper.
2. In a mixing bowl, combine almond flour, cocoa powder, baking powder, and salt.
3. In a separate bowl, whisk together melted butter, sweetener, eggs, and vanilla extract until smooth.
4. Fold the dry ingredients into the wet mixture gradually until they are well blended. Stir in dark chocolate chips if desired.
5. Pour the batter into the prepared pan and spread evenly.
6. A toothpick inserted in the center should come out with a few moist crumbs after baking for 18 to 20 minutes.
7. Allow to cool before slicing into squares.

Nutritional value per serving: Calories: 170, Carbs: 5g, Fiber: 2g, Sugars: 1g, Protein: 4g, Saturated fat: 7g, Unsaturated fat: 4g

Difficulty rating: ★★☆☆☆

Tips for ingredient variations: Add chopped nuts or a drizzle of sugar-free caramel for a flavor twist.

Coconut Fat Bombs

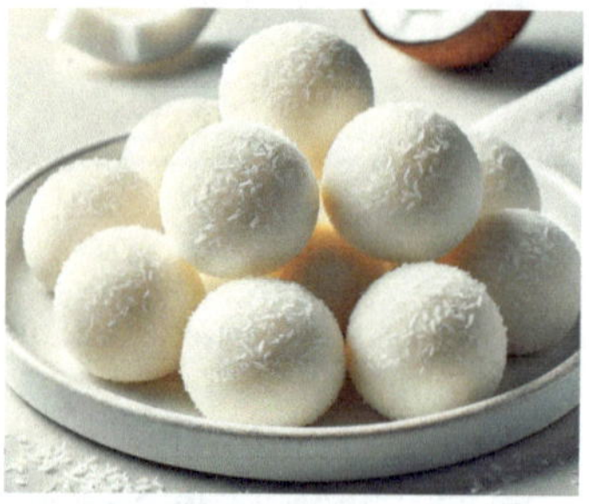

Number of servings: 12
Preparation time: 10 minutes
Cooking time: 0 minutes

Ingredients:

- 1/2 cup coconut oil, melted
- 1/2 cup unsweetened shredded coconut
- 2 tbsp almond butter
- 2 tbsp powdered erythritol or stevia
- 1 tsp vanilla extract

Directions:

1. In a mixing bowl, combine melted coconut oil, shredded coconut, almond butter, sweetener, and vanilla extract.
2. Stir until well mixed and smooth.
3. Spoon the mixture into silicone molds or mini muffin cups.
4. Freeze for at least 30 minutes until firm.
5. Store in the freezer and enjoy as needed.

Nutritional value per serving: Calories: 90, Carbs: 1g, Fiber: 1g, Sugars: 0g, Protein: 1g, Saturated fat: 7g, Unsaturated fat: 1g

Difficulty rating: ★☆☆☆☆

Tips for ingredient variations: Add a pinch of cocoa powder or cinnamon for an extra kick.

Low-Carb Cheesecake Cups

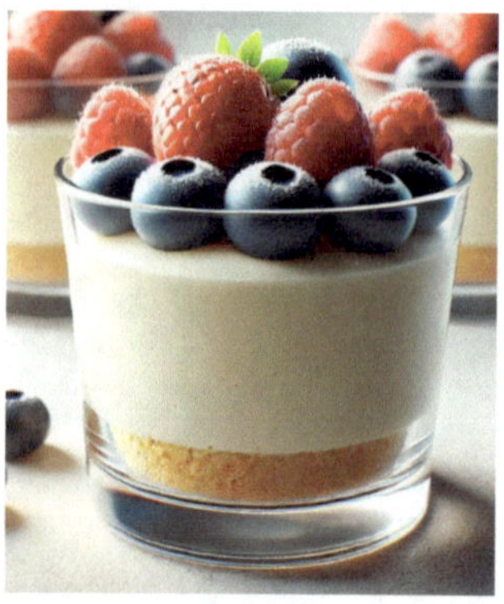

Number of servings: 6
Preparation time: 10 minutes
Cooking time: 0 minutes

Ingredients:

- 8 oz cream cheese, softened
- 1/4 cup powdered erythritol or stevia
- 1 tsp vanilla extract
- 1/2 cup heavy cream, whipped
- Fresh berries for topping

Directions:

1. In a mixing bowl, beat the cream cheese, sweetener, and vanilla extract until smooth.
2. Gently fold in the whipped heavy cream until combined.
3. Spoon the cheesecake mixture into serving cups.
4. Top with fresh berries and chill for at least 1 hour before serving.

Nutritional value per serving: Calories: 190, Carbs: 4g, Fiber: 1g, Sugars: 2g, Protein: 3g, Saturated fat: 10g, Unsaturated fat: 2g

Difficulty rating: ★☆☆☆☆

Tips for ingredient variations: Top with a dollop of sugar-free chocolate syrup or crushed nuts.

Vanilla Chia Seed Pudding

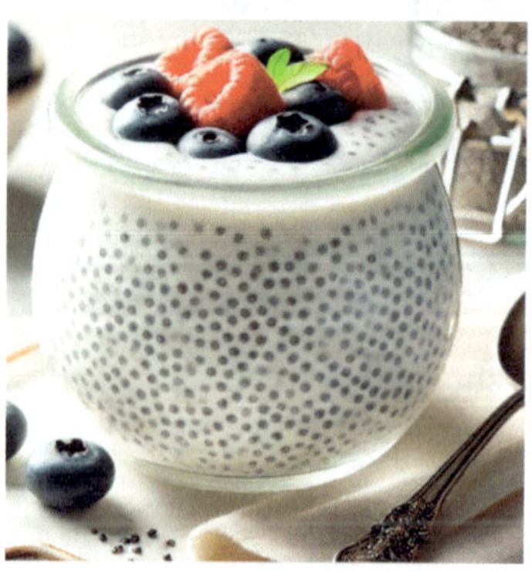

Number of servings: 2
Preparation time: 5 minutes
Cooking time: 0 minutes (overnight chilling)

Ingredients:

- 1/2 cup unsweetened almond milk
- 2 tbsp chia seeds
- 1 tsp vanilla extract
- 1 tbsp powdered erythritol or stevia
- Fresh berries for topping (optional)

Directions:

1. In a mixing bowl, whisk together almond milk, chia seeds, vanilla extract, and sweetener.
2. Transfer the mixture to a jar or container and refrigerate for at least 4 hours, preferably overnight, until thickened.
3. Stir before serving and top with fresh berries if desired.

Nutritional value per serving: Calories: 100, Carbs: 3g, Fiber: 2g, Sugars: 0g, Protein: 3g, Saturated fat: 0g, Unsaturated fat: 1g

Difficulty rating: ★☆☆☆☆

Tips for ingredient variations: Mix in a pinch of cinnamon or a splash of coconut milk for added flavor.

Peanut Butter Protein Balls

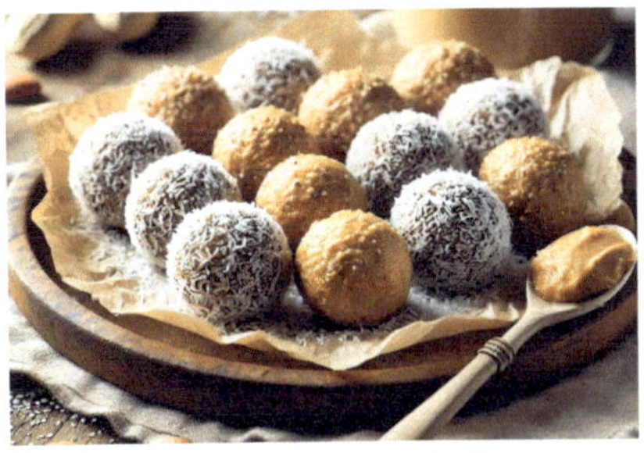

Number of servings: 12 balls
Preparation time: 10 minutes
Cooking time: 0 minutes

Ingredients:

- 1/2 cup natural peanut butter (no sugar added)
- 1/4 cup almond flour
- 2 tbsp unsweetened shredded coconut
- 2 tbsp chia seeds
- 1 tbsp cocoa powder (optional)
- 1-2 tbsp low-carb sweetener (erythritol or stevia)
- 1/4 cup unsweetened almond milk (as needed)

Directions:

1. In a medium bowl, combine peanut butter, almond flour, shredded coconut, chia seeds, and cocoa powder.
2. Add the sweetener and mix well. Gradually add almond milk, one tablespoon at a time, until the mixture comes together into a dough-like consistency.
3. Roll the mixture into 12 equal-sized balls and place them on a plate or tray lined with parchment paper.
4. Refrigerate for 20-30 minutes until firm.
5. Store in an airtight container in the refrigerator for up to one week.

Nutritional value per ball: Calories: 90, Carbs: 3g, Fiber: 1g, Sugars: 1g, Protein: 4g, Saturated fat: 1g, Unsaturated fat: 5g

Difficulty rating: ★☆☆☆☆

Tips for ingredient variations: Substitute almond flour with coconut flour for a slightly sweeter taste or add crushed nuts for texture.

Berries with Coconut Cream

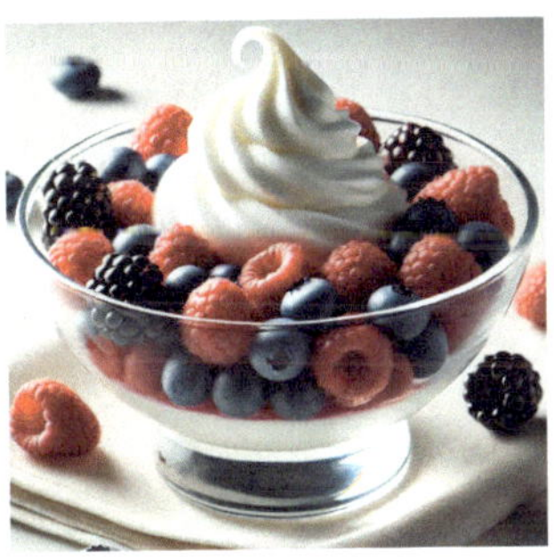

Number of servings: 2
Preparation time: 5 minutes
Cooking time: 0 minutes

Ingredients:

- 1 cup mixed berries (blueberries, raspberries, strawberries)
- 1/2 cup coconut cream (chilled)
- 1 tsp vanilla extract
- 1-2 tsp low-carb sweetener (optional)

Directions:

1. Divide the berries evenly into two serving bowls.
2. In a separate bowl, whisk the chilled coconut cream with vanilla extract and sweetener until smooth and slightly whipped.
3. Spoon the coconut cream over the berries.
4. Serve immediately for a light and refreshing dessert.

Nutritional value per serving: Calories: 120, Carbs: 6g, Fiber: 2g, Sugars: 4g, Protein: 1g, Saturated fat: 9g, Unsaturated fat: 1g

Difficulty rating: ★☆☆☆☆

Tips for ingredient variations: Top with crushed nuts or a sprinkle of cinnamon for added flavor.

Chocolate Avocado Mousse

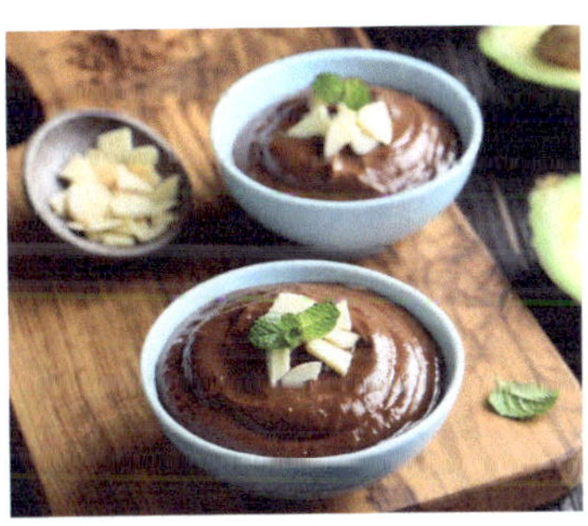

Number of servings: 2
Preparation time: 5 minutes
Cooking time: 0 minutes

Ingredients:

- 1 ripe avocado
- 2 tbsp unsweetened cocoa powder
- 2 tbsp unsweetened almond milk
- 1-2 tbsp low-carb sweetener (erythritol or monk fruit)
- 1 tsp vanilla extract
- Pinch of sea salt

Directions:

1. Scoop the avocado flesh into a blender or food processor.
2. Add sea salt, vanilla extract, sweetener, almond milk, and chocolate powder. Blend until smooth and creamy.
3. Divide the mousse into two small bowls or glasses.
4. Chill in the refrigerator for 10-15 minutes before serving.

Nutritional value per serving: Calories: 160, Carbs: 8g, Fiber: 4g, Sugars: 2g, Protein: 2g, Saturated fat: 2g, Unsaturated fat: 13g

Difficulty rating: ★☆☆☆☆

Tips for ingredient variations: Top with a dollop of whipped coconut cream or sprinkle with chopped nuts for extra texture.

Almond Butter Cookies

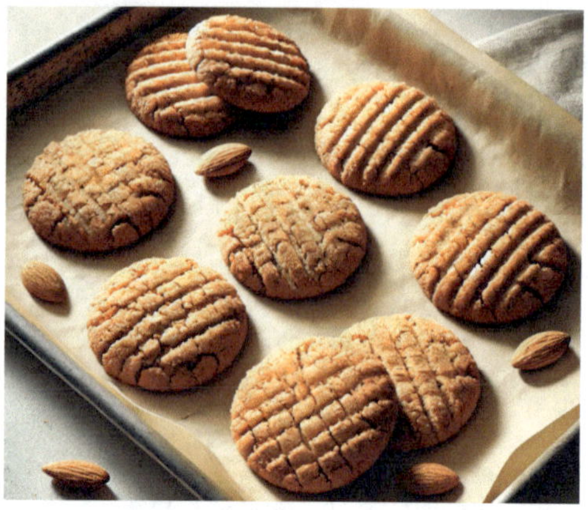

Number of servings: 12 cookies

Preparation time: 10 minutes

Cooking time: 12 minutes

Ingredients:

- 1 cup almond butter (no sugar added)
- 1 large egg
- 1/4 cup low-carb sweetener (erythritol or stevia)
- 1 tsp vanilla extract
- 1/2 tsp baking powder

Directions:

1. Preheat the oven to 350°F (175°C) and line a baking sheet with parchment paper.
2. In a mixing bowl, combine almond butter, egg, sweetener, vanilla extract, and baking powder until smooth.
3. Place the dough on the baking sheet after rolling it into 12 little balls. Flatten each ball slightly with a fork.
4. Bake for 10-12 minutes or until the edges are golden.
5. Allow to cool completely before serving.

Nutritional value per cookie: Calories: 110, Carbs: 4g, Fiber: 1g, Sugars: 1g, Protein: 4g, Saturated fat: 1g, Unsaturated fat: 9g

Difficulty rating: ★☆☆☆☆

Tips for ingredient variations: Sprinkle with a pinch of sea salt or add dark chocolate chips (sugar-free) for extra flavor.

Lemon Coconut Bars

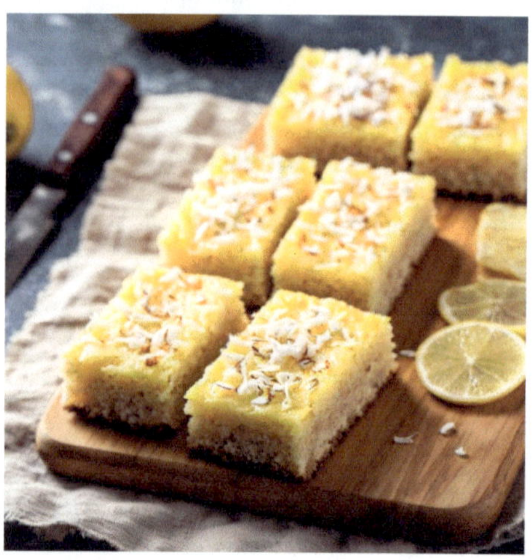

Number of servings: 8 bars

Preparation time: 10 minutes

Cooking time: 15 minutes

Ingredients:

- 1 cup almond flour
- 1/4 cup unsweetened shredded coconut
- 2 tbsp coconut oil, melted
- 1 tbsp low-carb sweetener (erythritol or monk fruit)
- Zest and juice of 1 lemon
- 2 large eggs
- 1/4 cup coconut cream

Directions:

1. Preheat the oven to 350°F (175°C) and line an 8x8-inch baking dish with parchment paper.
2. In a bowl, mix almond flour, shredded coconut, coconut oil, and sweetener until crumbly. Press the mixture into the bottom of the baking dish.
3. Bake the crust for 8 minutes until lightly golden.
4. Meanwhile, whisk together the eggs, lemon zest, lemon juice, sweetener, and coconut cream in a bowl.
5. Pour the lemon mixture over the baked crust and return to the oven for 10-12 minutes until set.
6. Cool completely before slicing into bars.

Nutritional value per bar: Calories: 150, Carbs: 5g, Fiber: 2g, Sugars: 2g, Protein: 3g, Saturated fat: 9g, Unsaturated fat: 3g

Difficulty rating: ★★☆☆☆

Tips for ingredient variations: Garnish with extra shredded coconut or a sprinkle of powdered erythritol for a decorative touch.

Low-Carb Ice Cream (Almond Milk-Based)

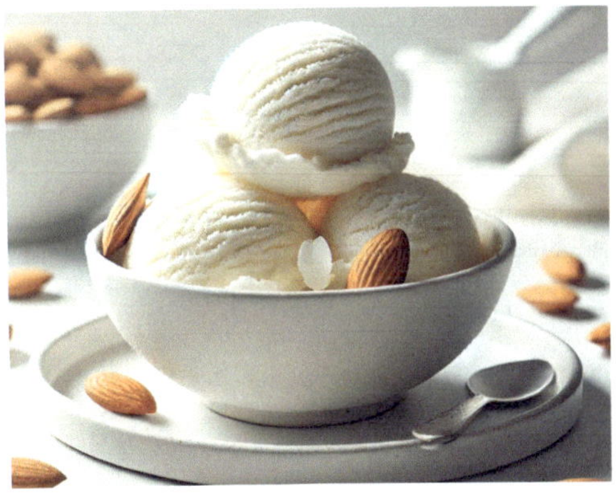

Number of servings: 4

Preparation time: 10 minutes

Cooking time: 0 minutes (plus 4 hours freezing time)

Ingredients:

- 2 cups unsweetened almond milk
- 1/2 cup heavy cream
- 1/3 cup low-carb sweetener (like erythritol or stevia)
- 1 tsp vanilla extract
- Pinch of sea salt

Directions:

1. In a mixing bowl, combine almond milk, heavy cream, sweetener, vanilla extract, and sea salt. Whisk until fully incorporated.
2. As directed by the manufacturer, pour the ingredients into an ice cream machine and churn.
3. If you don't have an ice cream maker, pour the mixture into a shallow container, freeze for 4 hours, and stir every 30 minutes to break up ice crystals.
4. Once frozen, scoop and serve immediately.

Nutritional value per serving: Calories: 90, Carbs: 3g, Fiber: 0g, Sugars: 1g, Protein: 2g, Saturated fat: 4g, Unsaturated fat: 2g

Difficulty rating: ★☆☆☆☆

Tips for ingredient variations: Add sugar-free chocolate chips or a swirl of unsweetened cocoa powder for a flavor twist.

Cinnamon Almond Muffins with Cream Cheese Frosting

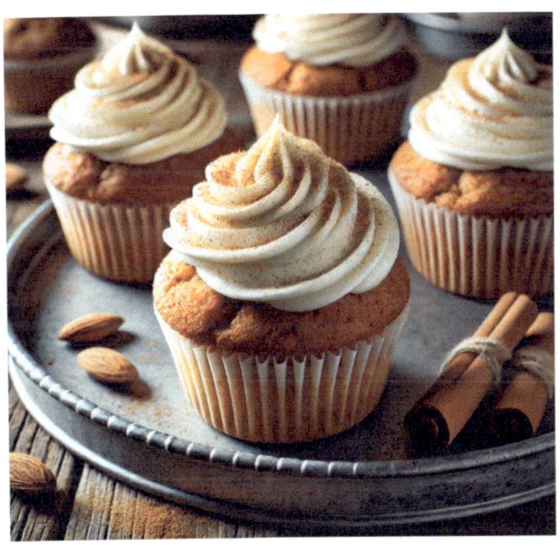

Number of servings: 12 muffins

Preparation time: 10 minutes

Cooking time: 20 minutes

Ingredients for Muffins:

- 2 cups almond flour
- 1/3 cup low-carb sweetener
- 1 tsp baking powder
- 1 tsp cinnamon
- 3 large eggs
- 1/3 cup unsweetened almond milk
- 1 tsp vanilla extract

Ingredients for Frosting:

- 4 oz cream cheese, softened
- 2 tbsp butter, softened
- 2 tbsp low-carb sweetener
- 1/2 tsp vanilla extract

Directions:

1. Preheat the oven to 350°F (175°C) and line a muffin tin with paper liners.
2. In a large bowl, mix almond flour, sweetener, baking powder, and cinnamon.
3. In a separate bowl, whisk eggs, almond milk, and vanilla extract. Gradually combine wet and dry ingredients until a smooth batter forms.
4. Spoon the batter evenly into the muffin cups.
5. Bake for 18-20 minutes or until a toothpick inserted comes out clean. Let cool completely.
6. For the frosting, beat together cream cheese, butter, sweetener, and vanilla extract until smooth. Spread or pipe onto cooled muffins.

Nutritional value per serving (with frosting): Calories: 150, Carbs: 4g, Fiber: 2g, Sugars: 1g, Protein: 6g, Saturated fat: 5g, Unsaturated fat: 3g

Difficulty rating: ★★☆☆☆

Tips for ingredient variations: Add a sprinkle of chopped walnuts to the batter for added texture and flavor.

Cinnamon Roll Fat Bombs

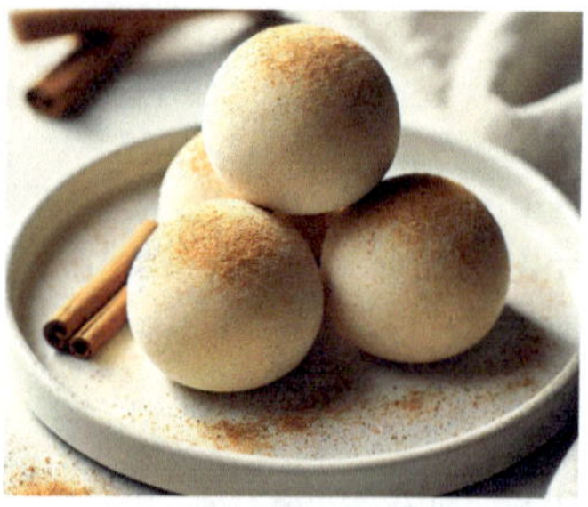

Number of servings: 12
Preparation time: 10 minutes
Cooking time: 0 minutes

Ingredients:

- 1/2 cup almond butter
- 1/4 cup unsweetened shredded coconut
- 2 tbsp coconut oil, melted
- 1/4 cup low-carb sweetener
- 1 tsp cinnamon
- 1 tsp vanilla extract

Directions:

1. In a mixing bowl, combine almond butter, shredded coconut, coconut oil, sweetener, cinnamon, and vanilla extract. Mix until smooth.
2. Roll the mixture into 12 small balls and place them on a parchment-lined tray.
3. Refrigerate for 30 minutes until firm.
4. Store in an airtight container in the fridge for up to 1 week.

Nutritional value per serving: Calories: 110, Carbs: 3g, Fiber: 1g, Sugars: 1g, Protein: 3g, Saturated fat: 4g, Unsaturated fat: 6g

Difficulty rating: ★☆☆☆☆

Tips for ingredient variations: Drizzle with melted sugar-free chocolate for an extra treat.

Raspberry Cheesecake Bites

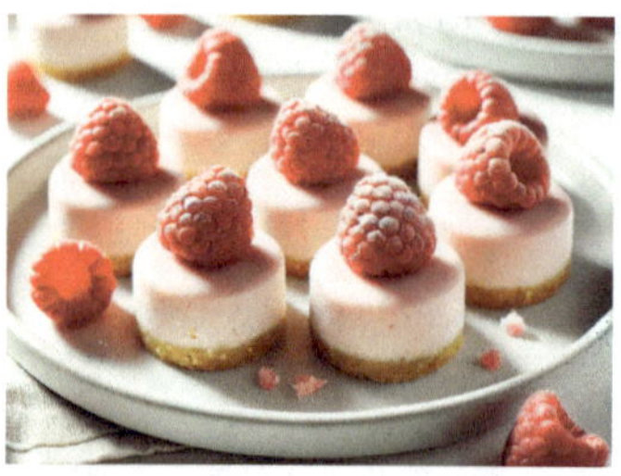

Number of servings: 8 bites
Preparation time: 15 minutes
Cooking time: 0 minutes (plus 1 hour chilling time)

Ingredients:

- 8 oz cream cheese, softened
- 1/4 cup low-carb sweetener
- 1/2 tsp vanilla extract
- 1/4 cup fresh raspberries
- 1/4 cup almond flour (for crust, optional)
- 1 tbsp butter, melted (optional)

Directions:

1. If making a crust, mix almond flour and melted butter. Press a small amount into the bottom of silicone molds or mini muffin tins. Chill in the fridge for 10 minutes.
2. In a bowl, beat cream cheese, sweetener, and vanilla extract until smooth.
3. Gently fold in fresh raspberries.
4. Spoon the mixture onto the crust or directly into molds. Smooth the tops with a spoon.
5. Chill for at least 1 hour before serving.

Nutritional value per serving (without crust): Calories: 100, Carbs: 2g, Fiber: 0g, Sugars: 1g, Protein: 3g, Saturated fat: 6g, Unsaturated fat: 2g

Difficulty rating: ★☆☆☆☆

Tips for ingredient variations: Top with a sprinkle of crushed sugar-free chocolate or coconut flakes.

Chocolate Protein Mug Cake

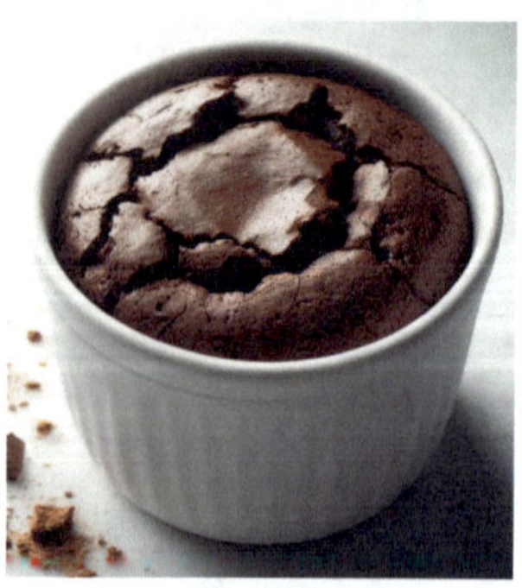

Number of servings: 1
Preparation time: 5 minutes
Cooking time: 1 minute

Ingredients:

- 2 tbsp almond flour
- 1 tbsp unsweetened cocoa powder
- 1 scoop chocolate protein powder
- 1/2 tsp baking powder
- 1 large egg
- 2 tbsp almond milk
- 1 tsp low-carb sweetener

Directions:

1. Combine the almond flour, baking powder, protein powder, and cocoa powder microwave-safe mug.
2. Add the egg, almond milk, and sweetener. Mix thoroughly until a smooth batter forms.
3. Microwave on high for 60-90 seconds until the cake is cooked through but still moist.
4. Let cool slightly before enjoying directly from the mug.

Nutritional value per serving: Calories: 190, Carbs: 5g, Fiber: 2g, Sugars: 1g, Protein: 15g, Saturated fat: 3g, Unsaturated fat: 4g

Difficulty rating: ★☆☆☆☆

Tips for ingredient variations: Add a dollop of sugar-free whipped cream or a drizzle of almond butter for extra indulgence.

60-Day Low Carb High Protein Meal Plan

Week 1

Day 1

- **Breakfast:** Scrambled Eggs with Spinach and Feta
- **Lunch:** Grilled Chicken Salad with Avocado and Olive Oil Dressing
- **Dinner:** Garlic Butter Salmon with Green Beans
- **Snack:** Almonds, Pecans, and Pumpkin Seed Mix

Day 2

- **Breakfast:** Greek Yogurt with Chia Seeds and Berries
- **Lunch:** Beef and Veggie Stir-Fry
- **Dinner:** Chicken Alfredo with Zoodles
- **Snack:** Cheese Crisps

Day 3

- **Breakfast:** Avocado and Smoked Salmon Toast
- **Lunch:** Zucchini Lasagna with Ricotta and Ground Turkey
- **Dinner:** Herb-Crusted Pork Chops with Mashed Cauliflower
- **Snack:** Celery Sticks with Peanut Butter

Day 4

- **Breakfast:** Mushroom and Cheese Omelette
- **Lunch:** Grilled Salmon with Steamed Broccoli
- **Dinner:** Thai Green Curry with Chicken and Zucchini
- **Snack:** Spicy Roasted Chickpeas with Turmeric

Day 5

- **Breakfast:** Protein Pancakes (made with almond flour)
- **Lunch:** Pulled Pork Salad Bowl
- **Dinner:** Garlic Parmesan Pork Tenderloin with Roasted Veggies
- **Snack:** Cottage Cheese with Paprika

Day 6

- **Breakfast:** Hard-Boiled Eggs with Avocado Slices
- **Lunch:** Tuna Salad Lettuce Wraps
- **Dinner:** Chili Lime Shrimp with Sautéed Peppers
- **Snack:** Deviled Eggs with Avocado

Day 7

- **Breakfast:** Sausage and Egg Breakfast Bowl
- **Lunch:** Low-Carb Turkey Chili
- **Dinner:** Broiled Steak with Chimichurri Sauce and Grilled Asparagus
- **Snack:** Berries with Coconut Cream

Week 2

Day 1

- **Breakfast:** Zucchini Noodles with Fried Egg and Parmesan
- **Lunch:** BLT Lettuce Wraps
- **Dinner:** Keto-Friendly Meatloaf with Cauliflower Rice
- **Snack:** Hard-Boiled Eggs with Mustard

Day 2

- **Breakfast:** Almond Butter Smoothie
- **Lunch:** Spinach and Tuna Salad with Lemon Dressing
- **Dinner:** Grilled Lamb Chops with Spinach Salad
- **Snack:** Low-Carb Trail Mix

Day 3

- **Breakfast:** Chia Pudding with Vanilla and Coconut Milk
- **Lunch:** Turkey Meatballs with Tomato Sauce
- **Dinner:** Grilled Swordfish with Lemon Butter Sauce
- **Snack:** Guacamole with Bell Pepper Slices

Day 4

- **Breakfast:** Turkey Bacon and Egg Cups
- **Lunch:** Egg Salad with Low-Carb Crackers
- **Dinner:** Shrimp Scampi with Spaghetti Squash
- **Snack:** Sliced Cucumber with Cream Cheese

Day 5

- **Breakfast:** Low-Carb Granola with Greek Yogurt
- **Lunch:** Steak Salad with Blue Cheese Crumbles
- **Dinner:** Low-Carb Beef Tacos in Lettuce Wraps
- **Snack:** Zucchini Chips

Day 6

- **Breakfast:** Cottage Cheese with Cucumber and Cherry Tomatoes
- **Lunch:** Baked Cod with Asparagus
- **Dinner:** Roasted Chicken Drumsticks with Zucchini Fries
- **Snack:** Almond Butter Cookies

Day 7

- **Breakfast:** Keto Waffles (almond flour and cream cheese-based)
- **Lunch:** Cauliflower Fried Rice with Chicken
- **Dinner:** Low-Carb Chicken Parmesan
- **Snack:** Dark Chocolate Mousse

Week 3

Day 1

- **Breakfast:** Spinach and Ricotta Breakfast Bake
- **Lunch:** Low-Carb Chicken Wraps (using lettuce or collard greens)
- **Dinner:** Roasted Duck Breast with Spinach and Mushrooms
- **Snack:** Turkey Jerky

Day 2

- **Breakfast:** Bell Pepper and Cheese Mini Frittatas
- **Lunch:** Caprese Salad with Grilled Chicken
- **Dinner:** Spaghetti Squash Carbonara
- **Snack:** Guacamole with Bell Pepper Slices

Day 3

- **Breakfast:** Protein Shake with Peanut Butter and Cocoa
- **Lunch:** Zoodles (Zucchini Noodles) with Pesto and Grilled Shrimp
- **Dinner:** Grilled Swordfish with Lemon Butter Sauce
- **Snack:** Almond Butter Cookies

Day 4

- **Breakfast:** Cottage Cheese with Cucumber and Cherry Tomatoes
- **Lunch:** Grilled Salmon with Steamed Broccoli
- **Dinner:** Herb-Crusted Pork Chops with Cauliflower Puree
- **Snack:** Cheese Crisps

Day 5

- **Breakfast:** Keto Waffles (almond flour and cream cheese-based)
- **Lunch:** Chicken Caesar Salad (without croutons)
- **Dinner:** Chili Lime Shrimp with Sautéed Peppers
- **Snack:** Celery Sticks with Peanut Butter

Day 6

- **Breakfast:** Low-Carb Breakfast Burrito (with egg wrap)
- **Lunch:** Egg Salad with Low-Carb Crackers
- **Dinner:** Garlic Butter Salmon with Green Beans
- **Snack:** Berries with Coconut Cream

Day 7

- **Breakfast:** Turkey Bacon and Egg Cups
- **Lunch:** Greek Salad with Feta and Grilled Chicken
- **Dinner:** Low-Carb Beef Tacos (with lettuce wraps)
- **Snack:** Zucchini Chips

Week 4

Day 1

- **Breakfast:** Chia Pudding with Vanilla and Coconut Milk
- **Lunch:** Pulled Pork Salad Bowl
- **Dinner:** Broiled Steak with Chimichurri Sauce
- **Snack:** Spicy Roasted Chickpeas with Turmeric

Day 2

- **Breakfast:** Almond Butter Smoothie
- **Lunch:** Spinach and Tuna Salad with Lemon Dressing
- **Dinner:** Keto-Friendly Meatloaf with Cauliflower Rice
- **Snack:** Low-Carb Trail Mix

Day 3

- **Breakfast:** Hard-Boiled Eggs with Avocado Slices
- **Lunch:** Turkey Meatballs with Tomato Sauce
- **Dinner:** Thai Green Curry with Chicken and Zucchini
- **Snack:** Deviled Eggs with Avocado

Day 4

- **Breakfast:** Cottage Cheese with Cucumber and Cherry Tomatoes
- **Lunch:** Steak Salad with Blue Cheese Crumbles
- **Dinner:** Grilled Lamb Chops with Spinach Salad
- **Snack:** Sliced Cucumber with Cream Cheese

Day 5

- **Breakfast:** Protein Pancakes (made with almond flour)
- **Lunch:** BLT Lettuce Wraps
- **Dinner:** Garlic Parmesan Pork Tenderloin with Roasted Veggies
- **Snack:** Cheese Crisps

Day 6

- **Breakfast:** Zucchini Noodles with Fried Egg and Parmesan
- **Lunch:** Baked Cod with Asparagus
- **Dinner:** Low-Carb Shepherd's Pie (cauliflower topping)
- **Snack:** Almond Butter Cookies

Day 7

- **Breakfast:** Greek Yogurt with Chia Seeds and Berries
- **Lunch:** Cauliflower Fried Rice with Chicken
- **Dinner:** Grilled Swordfish with Lemon Butter Sauce
- **Snack:** Dark Chocolate Mousse

Week 5

Day 1

- **Breakfast:** Spinach and Ricotta Breakfast Bake
- **Lunch:** Tuna Salad Lettuce Wraps
- **Dinner:** Shrimp Scampi with Spaghetti Squash
- **Snack:** Turkey Jerky

Day 2

- **Breakfast:** Mushroom and Cheese Omelette
- **Lunch:** Zoodles (Zucchini Noodles) with Pesto and Grilled Shrimp
- **Dinner:** Herb-Crusted Pork Chops with Cauliflower Puree
- **Snack:** Guacamole with Bell Pepper Slices

Day 3

- **Breakfast:** Bell Pepper and Cheese Mini Frittatas
- **Lunch:** Pulled Pork Salad Bowl
- **Dinner:** Garlic Butter Salmon with Green Beans
- **Snack:** Cheese Crisps

Day 4

- **Breakfast:** Protein Shake with Peanut Butter and Cocoa
- **Lunch:** Greek Salad with Feta and Grilled Chicken
- **Dinner:** Chili Lime Shrimp with Sautéed Peppers
- **Snack:** Low-Carb Trail Mix

Day 5

- **Breakfast:** Keto Waffles (almond flour and cream cheese-based)
- **Lunch:** Steak Salad with Blue Cheese Crumbles
- **Dinner:** Roasted Duck Breast with Spinach and Mushrooms
- **Snack:** Celery Sticks with Peanut Butter

Day 6

- **Breakfast:** Cottage Cheese with Cucumber and Cherry Tomatoes
- **Lunch:** Grilled Salmon with Steamed Broccoli
- **Dinner:** Broiled Steak with Chimichurri Sauce
- **Snack:** Deviled Eggs with Avocado

Day 7

- **Breakfast:** Hard-Boiled Eggs with Avocado Slices
- **Lunch:** BLT Lettuce Wraps
- **Dinner:** Low-Carb Beef Tacos (with lettuce wraps)
- **Snack:** Zucchini Chips

Week 6

Day 1

- **Breakfast:** Chia Pudding with Vanilla and Coconut Milk
- **Lunch:** Grilled Chicken Salad with Avocado and Olive Oil Dressing
- **Dinner:** Herb-Crusted Pork Chops with Cauliflower Puree
- **Snack:** Cheese Crisps

Day 2

- **Breakfast:** Mushroom and Cheese Omelette
- **Lunch:** Tuna Salad Lettuce Wraps
- **Dinner:** Shrimp Scampi with Spaghetti Squash
- **Snack:** Spicy Roasted Chickpeas with Turmeric

Day 3

- **Breakfast:** Bell Pepper and Cheese Mini Frittatas
- **Lunch:** Spinach and Tuna Salad with Lemon Dressing
- **Dinner:** Broiled Steak with Chimichurri Sauce
- **Snack:** Low-Carb Trail Mix

Day 4

- **Breakfast:** Greek Yogurt with Chia Seeds and Berries
- **Lunch:** Zoodles (Zucchini Noodles) with Pesto and Grilled Shrimp
- **Dinner:** Grilled Swordfish with Lemon Butter Sauce
- **Snack:** Sliced Cucumber with Cream Cheese

Day 5

- **Breakfast:** Protein Pancakes (made with almond flour)
- **Lunch:** Egg Salad with Low-Carb Crackers
- **Dinner:** Garlic Butter Salmon with Green Beans
- **Snack:** Celery Sticks with Peanut Butter

Day 6

- **Breakfast:** Sausage and Egg Breakfast Bowl
- **Lunch:** Steak Salad with Blue Cheese Crumbles
- **Dinner:** Keto-Friendly Meatloaf with Cauliflower Rice
- **Snack:** Almond Butter Cookies

Day 7

- **Breakfast:** Spinach and Ricotta Breakfast Bake
- **Lunch:** Greek Salad with Feta and Grilled Chicken
- **Dinner:** Chili Lime Shrimp with Sautéed Peppers
- **Snack:** Deviled Eggs with Avocado

Week 7

Day 1

- **Breakfast:** Hard-Boiled Eggs with Avocado Slices
- **Lunch:** BLT Lettuce Wraps
- **Dinner:** Garlic Parmesan Pork Tenderloin with Roasted Veggies
- **Snack:** Zucchini Chips

Day 2

- **Breakfast:** Almond Butter Smoothie
- **Lunch:** Pulled Pork Salad Bowl
- **Dinner:** Herb-Crusted Pork Chops with Cauliflower Puree
- **Snack:** Cheese Crisps

Day 3

- **Breakfast:** Bell Pepper and Cheese Mini Frittatas
- **Lunch:** Egg Salad with Low-Carb Crackers
- **Dinner:** Grilled Swordfish with Lemon Butter Sauce
- **Snack:** Low-Carb Trail Mix

Day 4

- **Breakfast:** Cottage Cheese with Cucumber and Cherry Tomatoes
- **Lunch:** Spinach and Tuna Salad with Lemon Dressing
- **Dinner:** Chili Lime Shrimp with Sautéed Peppers
- **Snack:** Spicy Roasted Chickpeas with Turmeric

Day 5

- **Breakfast:** Greek Yogurt with Chia Seeds and Berries
- **Lunch:** Tuna Salad Lettuce Wraps
- **Dinner:** Low-Carb Chicken Parmesan
- **Snack:** Celery Sticks with Peanut Butter

Day 6

- **Breakfast:** Zucchini Noodles with Fried Egg and Parmesan
- **Lunch:** Greek Salad with Feta and Grilled Chicken
- **Dinner:** Shrimp Scampi with Spaghetti Squash
- **Snack:** Deviled Eggs with Avocado

Day 7

- **Breakfast:** Keto Waffles (almond flour and cream cheese-based)
- **Lunch:** Low-Carb Turkey Chili
- **Dinner:** Garlic Butter Salmon with Green Beans
- **Snack:** Almond Butter Cookies

Week 8

Day 1

- **Breakfast:** Protein Pancakes (made with almond flour)
- **Lunch:** Zoodles (Zucchini Noodles) with Pesto and Grilled Shrimp
- **Dinner:** Broiled Steak with Chimichurri Sauce
- **Snack:** Cheese Crisps

Day 2

- **Breakfast:** Almond Butter Smoothie
- **Lunch:** Greek Salad with Feta and Grilled Chicken
- **Dinner:** Grilled Swordfish with Lemon Butter Sauce
- **Snack:** Spicy Roasted Chickpeas with Turmeric

Day 3

- **Breakfast:** Sausage and Egg Breakfast Bowl
- **Lunch:** Pulled Pork Salad Bowl
- **Dinner:** Garlic Butter Salmon with Green Beans
- **Snack:** Zucchini Chips

Day 4

- **Breakfast:** Spinach and Ricotta Breakfast Bake
- **Lunch:** Egg Salad with Low-Carb Crackers
- **Dinner:** Herb-Crusted Pork Chops with Cauliflower Puree
- **Snack:** Low-Carb Trail Mix

Day 5

- **Breakfast:** Greek Yogurt with Chia Seeds and Berries
- **Lunch:** Spinach and Tuna Salad with Lemon Dressing
- **Dinner:** Shrimp Scampi with Spaghetti Squash
- **Snack:** Deviled Eggs with Avocado

Day 6

- **Breakfast:** Hard-Boiled Eggs with Avocado Slices
- **Lunch:** BLT Lettuce Wraps
- **Dinner:** Keto-Friendly Meatloaf with Cauliflower Rice
- **Snack:** Almond Butter Cookies

Day 7

- **Breakfast:** Mushroom and Cheese Omelette
- **Lunch:** Steak Salad with Blue Cheese Crumbles
- **Dinner:** Low-Carb Shepherd's Pie (cauliflower topping)
- **Snack:** Dark Chocolate Mousse

Week 9

Day 1

- **Breakfast:** Chia Pudding with Vanilla and Coconut Milk
- **Lunch:** Low-Carb Chicken Wraps (using lettuce or collard greens)
- **Dinner:** Grilled Lamb Chops with Spinach Salad
- **Snack:** Turkey Jerky

Day 2

- **Breakfast:** Almond Butter Smoothie
- **Lunch:** Zoodles (Zucchini Noodles) with Pesto and Grilled Shrimp
- **Dinner:** Herb-Crusted Pork Chops with Cauliflower Puree
- **Snack:** Spicy Roasted Chickpeas with Turmeric

Day 3

- **Breakfast:** Sausage and Egg Breakfast Bowl
- **Lunch:** Egg Salad with Low-Carb Crackers
- **Dinner:** Shrimp Scampi with Spaghetti Squash
- **Snack:** Cheese Crisps

Day 4

- **Breakfast:** Spinach and Ricotta Breakfast Bake
- **Lunch:** Greek Salad with Feta and Grilled Chicken
- **Dinner:** Broiled Steak with Chimichurri Sauce
- **Snack:** Low-Carb Trail Mix

Conclusion

A Path to Wellness: Summarizing the Benefits and Embracing the Journey

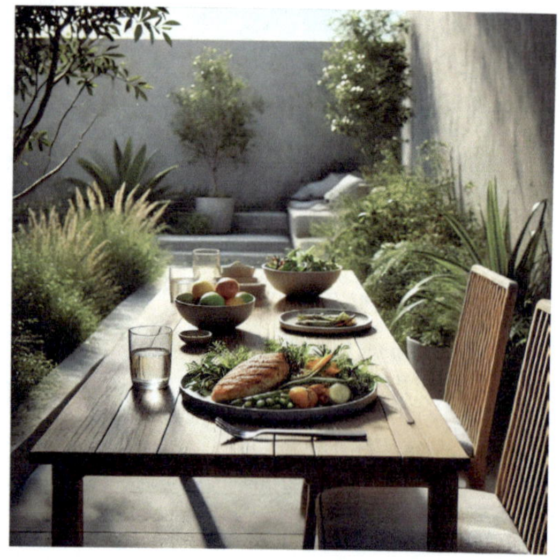

The LCHP lifestyle transcends the concept of dieting; it is a powerful shift toward sustainable health and vitality. This cookbook provides you with the essential tools, knowledge, and recipes to align effortlessly with your personal goals—whether focused on weight loss, boosting energy, or enhancing overall well-being. Embracing this journey means not only committing to a healthier version of yourself but also celebrating a way of life that prioritizes flavorful, nutrient-packed meals rooted in the principles shared here.

Beyond its impact on the scale, the LCHP diet offers profound health benefits. Reducing carbohydrate intake helps stabilize insulin levels, supports balanced blood sugar, and harnesses the body's natural ability to burn fat as a steady energy source, unlocking a new level of vitality.

Protein, the cornerstone of this approach, supports lean muscle maintenance, enhances metabolism, and keeps you feeling satisfied throughout the day. Meanwhile, healthy fats provide sustained energy and support cellular health, while the inclusion of low-glycemic vegetables ensures that your body receives essential vitamins, minerals, and fiber.

As you've discovered, the LCHP diet is more than a tool for physical transformation; it nurtures mental clarity, emotional balance, and a deeper connection with the food you consume. The recipes in this book demonstrate how simple ingredients can create dishes that are as enjoyable as they are nourishing. With every meal, you reinforce the positive habits that lead to long-term success.

A Call to Action: Taking the First Steps Toward Transformation

Your journey toward better health begins with a single step, and the path is yours to design. Start by incorporating one or two recipes from this book into your weekly routine. Let breakfast be your starting point, perhaps with a nutrient-packed spinach and mushroom omelet or almond flour pancakes that balance flavor and nutrition. As you grow comfortable, expand your repertoire, exploring vibrant salads, hearty mains, and indulgent desserts that stay true to the LCHP principles.

Set yourself up for success by organizing your pantry and planning your meals. The foundational principles in this book, paired with practical tips, make it easier than ever to stay consistent. Begin by stocking your kitchen with high-quality proteins, low-carb vegetables, and healthy fats. Experiment with spices and condiments to enhance the flavor of your dishes and keep your culinary journey exciting.

Consistency is key, but flexibility is equally important. Life is dynamic, and so should be your approach to eating. If a social occasion or unexpected challenge steers you temporarily away from the LCHP framework, remember that balance—not perfection—is the ultimate goal. The recipes and principles in this book are tools to guide you, not to restrict you.

To fully embrace this lifestyle, take time to reflect on the deeper reasons behind your commitment. Whether it's improving energy, achieving a specific health milestone, or simply feeling more vibrant each day, keep your goals at the forefront. Visualize the outcomes and celebrate the small victories along the way, knowing that each choice contributes to a bigger picture.

Ultimately, this journey is about empowerment rather than just food. You are making an investment in a happier, healthier future by taking charge of your diet. The recipes in this book serve as a foundation, but the real transformation happens in your kitchen, your habits, and your mindset. Start today, and let this be the beginning of a lifelong relationship with food that fuels your body, mind, and spirit.

Made in the USA
Columbia, SC
27 April 2025

57196546R00046